GOUT DIET COOKBOOK

by Henry Smith

© Copyright 2021 by Henry Smith - All rights reserved.

The following Book is reproduced below with the goal of providing information that is as accurate and reliable as possible. Regardless, purchasing this Book can be seen as consent to the fact that both the publisher and the author of this book are in no way experts on the topics discussed within and that any recommendations or suggestions that are made herein are for entertainment purposes only. Professionals should be consulted as needed prior to undertaking any of the actions endorsed herein.

This declaration is deemed fair and valid by both the American Bar Association and the Committee of Publishers Association and is legally binding throughout the United States.

Furthermore, the transmission, duplication, or reproduction of any of the following work including specific information will be considered an illegal act irrespective of if it is done electronically or in print. This extends to creating a secondary or tertiary copy of the work or a recorded copy and is only allowed with the express written consent from the Publisher. All additional rights reserved.

The information in the following pages is broadly considered a truthful and accurate account of facts and as such, any inattention, use, or misuse of the information in question by the reader will render any resulting actions solely under their purview. There are no scenarios in which the publisher or the original author of this work can be in any fashion deemed liable for any hardship or damages that may befall them after undertaking the information described herein.

Additionally, the information in the following pages is intended only for informational purposes and should thus be thought of as universal. As befitting its nature, it is presented without assurance regarding its prolonged validity or interim quality. Trademarks that are mentioned are done without written consent and can in no way be considered an endorsement from the trademark holder.

table of content

1   GOUT DIET COOKBOOK

3   TABLE OF CONTENT

5   INTRODUCTION TO GOUT DIET

7   PURINE TABLE INFORMATION

11   SMOOTHIE AND TEA

27   PASTA AND RICE

41   CHICKEN

61   FISH

table of content

1	GOUT DIET COOKBOOK	41	CHICKEN
3	TABLE OF CONTENT	42	CHICKEN AND VEGETABLE FRIED RICE
5	INTRODUCTION TO DIET	43	CHICKEN SALAD
7	TABLE	44	BROWN STEW CHICKEN
11	SMOOTHIE AND TEA	45	CHICKEN VEGGIE
12	AYURVEDIC TEA	46	CHICKEN-BROCCOLI STIR FRY
13	ROSEMARY TEA	48	CHICKEN WRAP
14	CINNAMON BLOSSOM TEA	49	CHICKEN WITH GARLIC AND SESAME
15	NETTLE AND BIRCH LEAF TEA	50	CHICKEN STROGANOFF
16	GOUT AND JOINT PAIN JUICE	51	LEMON AND ASPARAGUS CHICKEN
17	ANTI-INFLAMMATORY SMOOTHIE	53	CHICKEN CASSEROLE
18	VANILLA BLACK TEA SMOOTHIE	54	CHEESY CHICKEN BROCCOLI BAKE
19	PERSIMMON LASSI	55	ONE-PAN CHICKEN AND VEGGIES
20	COFFEE SMOOTHIE	56	CHICKEN WITH POTATOES
21	CHERRY "CHEESECAKE" SMOOTHIE	57	CHICKEN VEGETABLE SOUP
22	HEALTHY GREEN SHOT	58	CHICKEN AND LENTIL STEW
23	CHERRY CHOCOLATE SMOOTHIE	61	FISH
24	MANGO AND BANANA SMOOTHIE	63	SALMON ON FENNEL
27	PASTA AND RICE	64	STEAMED SNAPPA
28	ZUCCHINI SPAGHETTI	65	AVOCADO LIME SALMON
29	LENTIL NOODLES WITH PESTO	66	SOLE IN OVEN
30	GOAT CHEESE PASTA	67	BOILED SOLE
31	KONJAC PASTA WITH BERRIES	68	MACKEREL WITH GREEN SAUCE
32	SPAGHETTI WITH PAK CHOI	69	COD IN WHITE SAUCE
33	ZUCCHINI PASTA		
34	GOAT CHEESE RICE PAN		
35	COUSCOUS BASE RECIPE		
36	COUSCOUS WITH VEGETABLES		
37	COUSCOUS WITH ROSEMARY		
38	EASY RICE		
39	PASTA WITH EGGS		

GOUT DIET COOKBOOK

What is Gout?

Gout describes a set of conditions with one common feature – the accumulation of uric acid inside the joints. Uric acid is a product of the catabolic reaction of purine nucleotides, and it is a standard component of urine. Generally speaking, gout affects the joints of the feet and hands, causing edema (i.e., swelling), pain, and reduced range of motion.

The causes of gout

Gout stems from the buildup of uric acid in the bloodstream, which eventually leads to the leakage of this chemical into the joint capsules. (2) As a result, an inflammatory reaction sets in, producing the classic signs and symptoms of gout.

Researchers identified metabolic disorders, dehydration, and certain vascular diseases as potential triggers of uric acid accumulation. Additionally, medical conditions that affect the kidneys and thyroid also interfere with the body's ability to remove excess uric acid from the blood.

Other risk factors of gout include: (3)
Age – middle-aged men and postmenopausal women
Family history – having family members with gout increases the risk
Alcohol abuse – excessive alcohol consumption precipitates gout
Medication – diuretics, cyclosporine
Concurrent medical conditions – high blood pressure, thyroid disease, diabetes, kidney disease, and obstructive sleep apnea
Dietary choices – foods rich in gout-producing purines (e.g., some fish, organ meats, game meats). Foods that can trigger gout attacks
If you are susceptible to gout attacks, you need to avoid purine-producing foods. These foods typically contain more than 200 mg of purine per 3.5 ounces.

Here is a list of the significant purine-producing foods to avoid:
Fish: Herring, trout, mackerel, tuna, sardines, anchovies, haddock
Other seafood: Scallops, crab, shrimp, and roe
Organ meats: These include liver, kidneys, sweetbreads, and brain
Game meats: Examples include pheasant, veal, and venison, fatty meat broth or meat extracts, sausage, goose, duck, lard
Sugary beverages: Especially fruit juices and sugary sodas
Added sugars: honey, agave nectar, and high-fructose corn syrup
Yeasts: Nutritional yeast, brewer's yeast, and other yeast supplements
Alcohol specialty beer

A too restrictive diet also leads to a rise in uric acid concentration, derived from particular molecules' metabolism, called purines.
If you are overweight or obese, your diet should be moderately low-calorie to reach the desired weight gradually, but not excessively drastic to avoid causing a further increase in blood uric acid levels.

The general advice, beyond these first indications, are
Avoid prolonged fasting.
Avoid a diet too rich in fats and proteins, consequently avoiding or decreasing foods rich in purines (anchovies, brain, liver, kidneys, shrimp, sardines, ...).
Avoid alcohol consumption.
Drink plenty of water to prevent kidney stones from forming.
Consume copious amounts of fruits, vegetables, and whole grains, which provide healthy carbohydrates in complex form.

Following foods are good foods for GOUT diet:
plant foods: fruit, vegetables, nuts, seeds, including cereals, lean fish, chicken, turkey, skimmed milk, extra virgin olive oil, coffee, tea, and herbal teas.

Foods to consume with moderation:
mayonnaise, asparagus, peas, tomatoes, and spinach (limit to use these vegetables because of the suspect of relationship with the possibility of developing kidney stones, but a good intake of water allows their consumption), pork or beef (lean parts only), whole milk, dried fruit, simple sugars.

Another important trick is not to use too much fat when cooking, preferring approaches such as: steaming, boiling, plate, foil, sautéed.

If you want to consume a fry, you need to make sure that the oil temperature is high enough not to be absorbed by the food, but obviously, avoid fried foods in recent remission of an acute attack.

Instead of salt, use: garlic, onion, various spices, vinegar, lemon.

TABLE

Food with moderate purine mg/100g

Beef chuck, filet, fore rib, entrecote, shoulder, roast beef	120
Bean dry white seed	128
soya dry seed dry	190
chicken breast	175
chicken for roasting	115
chicken legs with skin and bone	110
fish anchovy	239
fish cod	109
fish haddock	139
fish herring roe	190
fish mackerel	145
fish redfish	241
fish salmon	170
fish sole	131
fish eel smoked	78
crayfish	60
ham cooked	131
grape dried raisin	107
lentil dry seed	127
linseed	105
lobster	118
peas chick, dry garbanzo seed	109
poppy seed	170
rabbit meat average	132

Food with low purine mg/100gr

almond	37	corn sweet	52
apple	14	cress	28
apricot	73	crispbread	60
asparagus	23	cucumber	7
aubergine	21	currant red	17
avocado	19	date dried	35
banana	57	elderberry black	33
bean sprouts	80	endive	17
bean french string beans haricot	37	fenel leaves	14
beans french dried	45	fig dried	64
blueberry, huckleberry, bilberry	22	grape	27
bread white	14	kale	48
broccoli	81	kiwi	18
brussels sprouts	69	leek	74
cabbage red savoy	35	lettuce	13
cabbage white	22	lettuce lambs	38
carrot	17	melon cantelope	33
cauliflower	51	mushroom chanterelle	17
celeriac	30	nuts brazil	23
cheese brie	7	nuts hazelnut	37
cheese cheddar ceshire	6	nuts peanut	79
cheese cottage	9	nuts walnut	25
cheese edam	7	oats whole grain	94
cheese Limburger	32	olive marinated green	29
cherry morelly	18	onion	13
cherry sweet	7	orange	19
chicory	12	parsley leaf	57
Chinese leaves	21	pasta made with eggs	40
chives	67	pea pod and seed, green	84

pea seed dry	95
peach	21
pear	12
peppers green	55
pineapple	19
plum	24
plum dried	64
potato	16
potato cooked with skin	18
pumpkin	44
radish	15
radishes	14
raspberry	18
rhubarb	12
rice white	26
rols bread	21
sauerkraut dripped off	16
sesame seeds	62
spinach	57
strawberry	21
tomato	11
yogurt 3.5 %fat	8

Reference: https://elevatehealthaz.com/wp-content/Purine%20Table.pdf

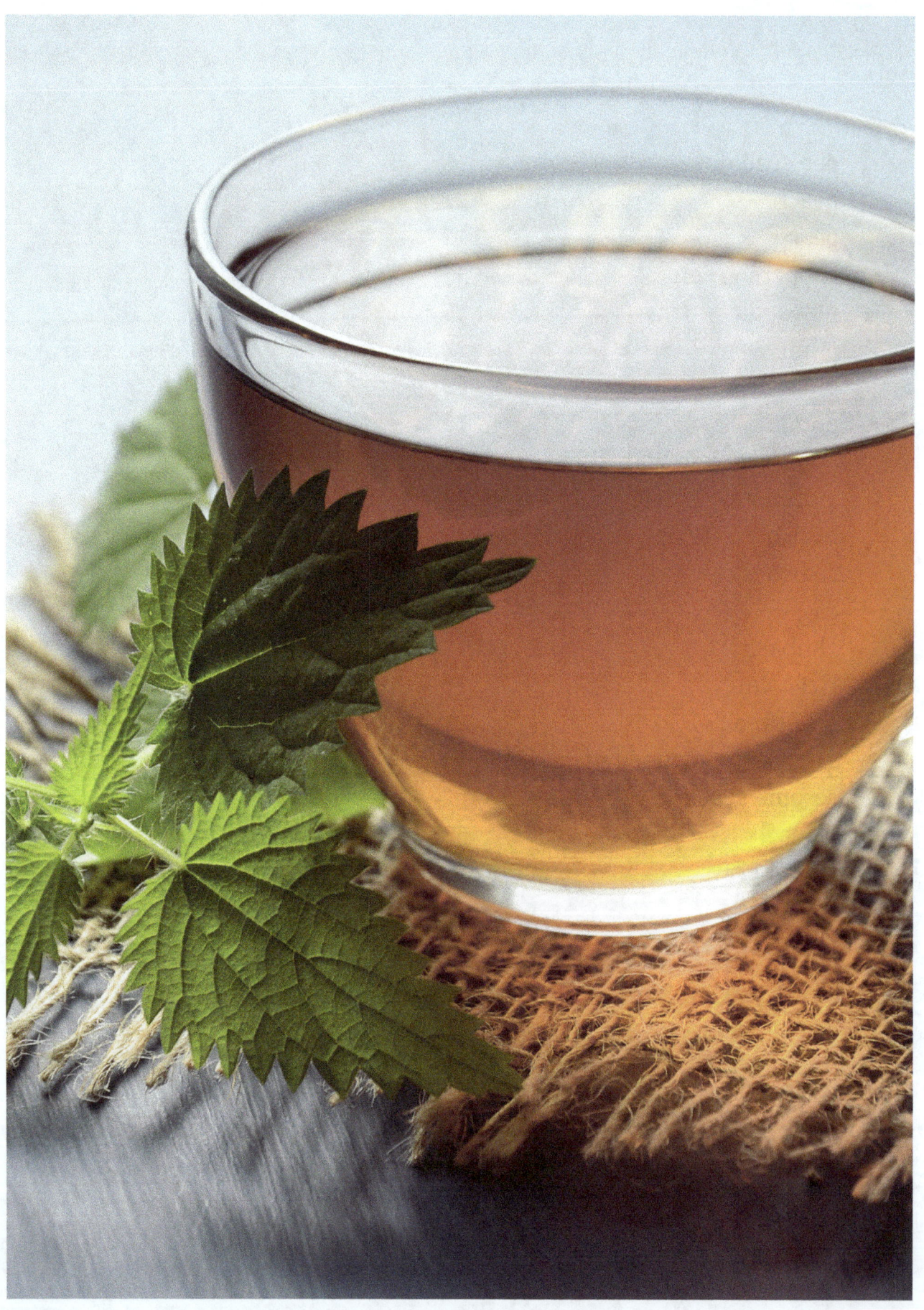

SMOOTHIE

TEA

 Servings: 4

 Calories: 5

 Ready in 10 min

AYURVEDIC TEA

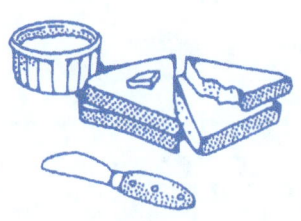

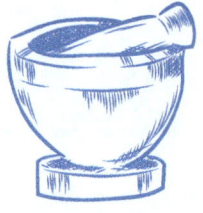

Ingredients:

1 tsp fennel seeds
1 tsp peppercorns
6 Cardamom capsules,
2 tbsp ginger root
2 garlic cloves
3 anise stars
1 piece of cinnamon
approx 0 mg purine

Instructions:

In a mortar, grind the pepper and fennel for a few seconds. Using the back of a knife, crack open the cardamom pod. Ginger should be washed and cut into small bits.
Toast the spices in a hot saucepan over medium heat for a few minutes. Bring to a boil with the ginger and around 35oz of water. Cook for approximately 25-30 minutes on low heat.
Divide the tea you made into four cups after draining it.

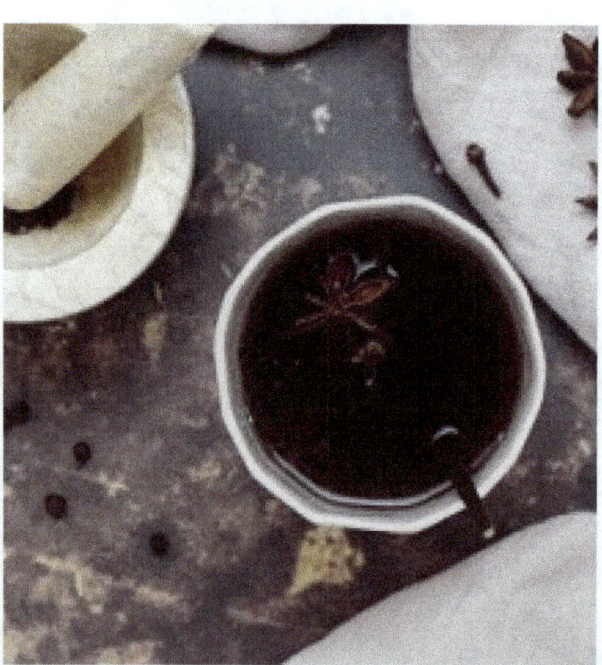

Servings:1

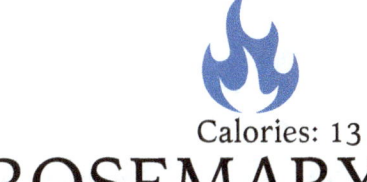
Calories: 13

ROSEMARY TEA

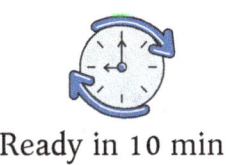
Ready in 10 min

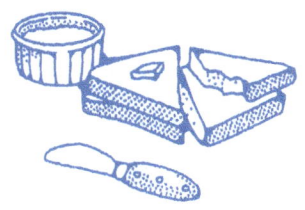

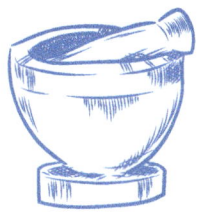

Ingredients:

1 rosemary branch
1 green tea bag
1 orange
approx 0 mg purine

Instructions:

Rinse the rosemary, shake it out, and put it in a mug.
Make a tea with the tea bag and 200 ml of water, as directed on the box, and top with the rosemary.
Take the orange and squeeze it.
Remove the teabag from the rosemary tea and stir in the orange juice.

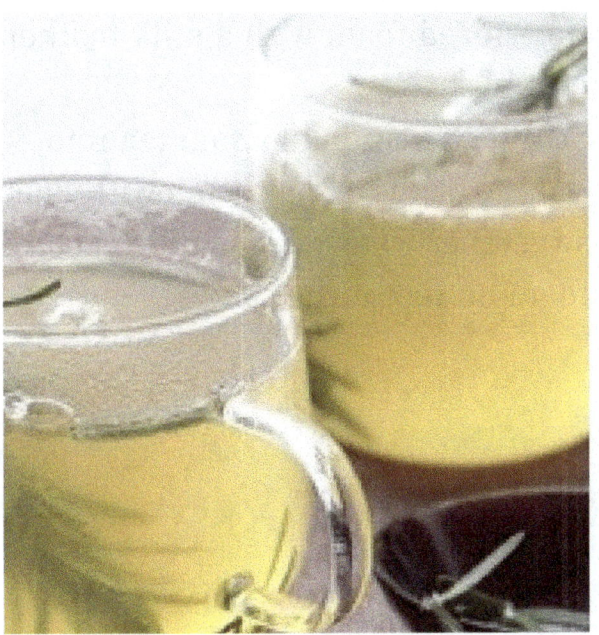

 Servings: 2    Calories: 29    Ready in 15min

CINNAMON BLOSSOM TEA

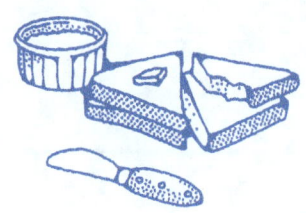   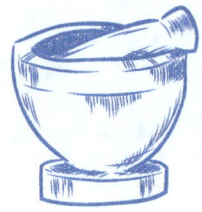

Ingredients:

1 cardamom pod
1 tsp cinnamon blossoms
1 tsp black tea or rooibos tea
8 tbsp Milk (1.5 percent fat; preferably long-life milk)
1 tsp cocoa powder (without sugar)
a liquid sweetener
approx 0 mg purine

Instructions:

In a small saucepan, bring the cinnamon blossoms, tea, cardamom, and 14oz water to a boil, then reduce to low heat and simmer for 8-10 minutes.
Meanwhile, warm the milk in a separate saucepan. Whisk in the cocoa powder and beat the mixture to a fine-pored foam with a milk frother or whisk.
Strain cinnamon blossom tea into mugs or cups and sweeten with liquid sweetener to taste. Place the cocoa foam on top of the cake.

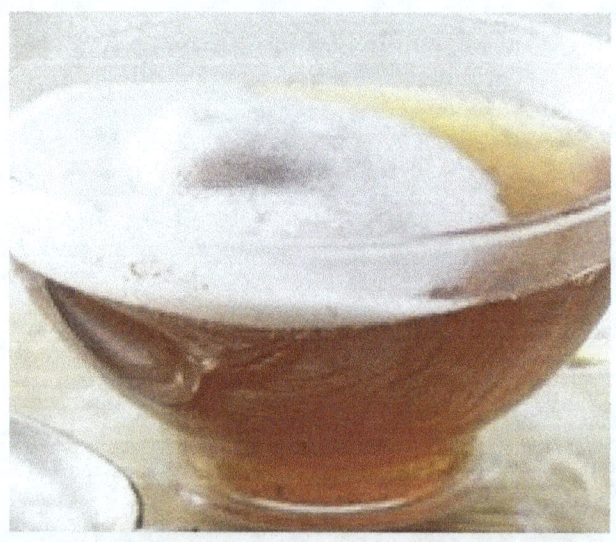

Servings: 1

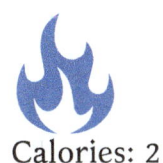
Calories: 2

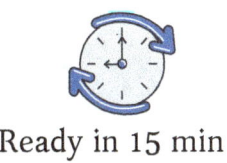
Ready in 15 min

NETTLE AND BIRCH LEAF TEA

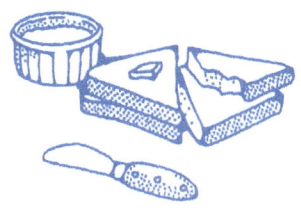

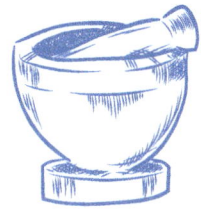

Ingredients:

2 tsp dried birch leaf
4 tsp dried nettle leaves
2 tsp dried juniper berry
1 lemon (organic)
approx 0 mg purine

Instructions:

Lightly mash the juniper berries in a mortar or with a big knife.
Combine nettle and birch leaves in a saucepan and add 1 cup of boiling water. Allow for an 8-minute rest period after covering.
While you're waiting, wash the lemon in hot water and pat it dry with a paper towel. Thinly peel the peel and cut it into fine strips with a peeler.
Strain the tea into a mug or glass using a sieve. Serve with lemon zest strips as a garnish.

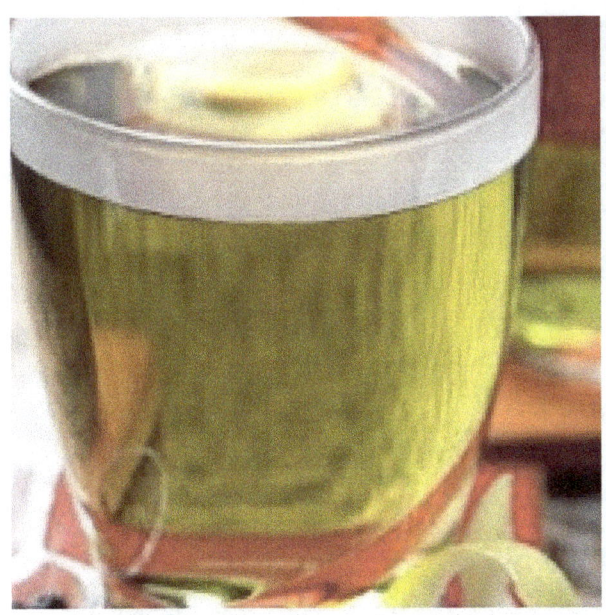

 Servings: 1

 Calories: 114

 Ready in 5 min

GOUT AND JOINT PAIN JUICE

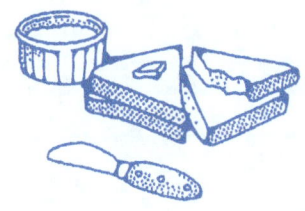

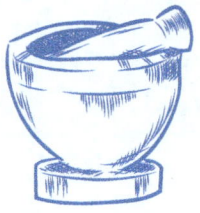

Ingredients:

Instructions:

half of a lemon
1-inch piece peeled ginger root
approx 0 mg purine

Run the ingredients through the juicer one by one. Drink the juice once a day.

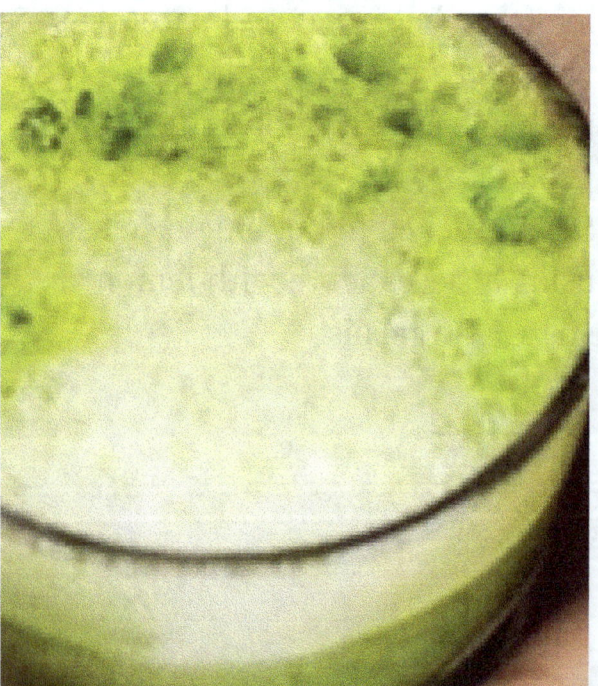

 Servings: 2

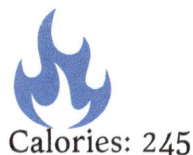 Calories: 245

 Ready in 5min

ANTI-INFLAMMATORY SMOOTHIE

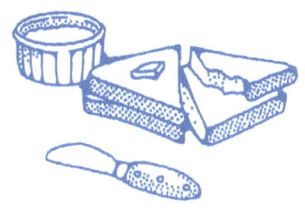

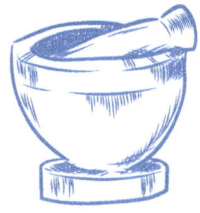

Ingredients:

1 cup Frozen Strawberries
½ can Coconut Milk
1 tsp ginger (fresh)
Cherry Juice (1-2 oz.) natural approx 10 mg purine

Instructions:

In a blender, add all ingredients and puree until smooth.

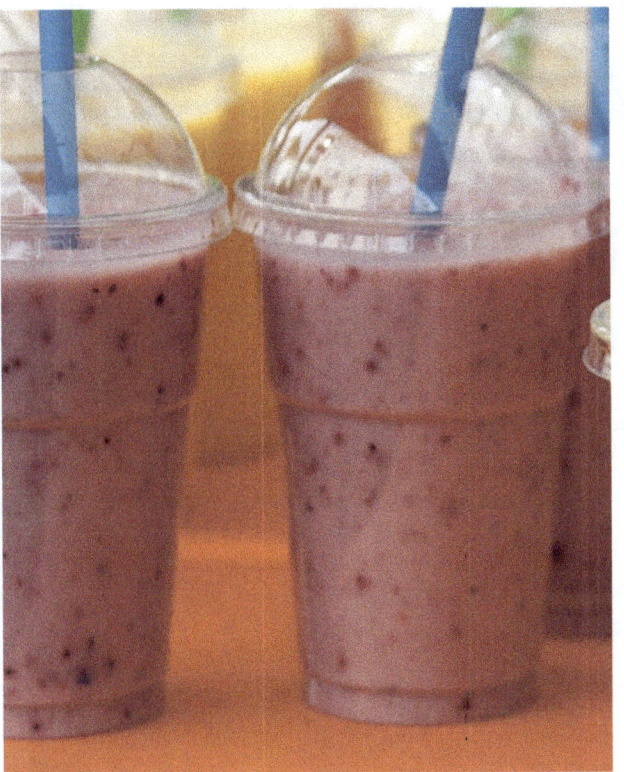

 Servings: 2 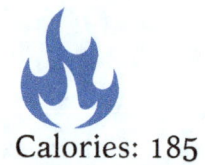 Calories: 185  Ready in 10 min

VANILLA BLACK TEA SMOOTHIE

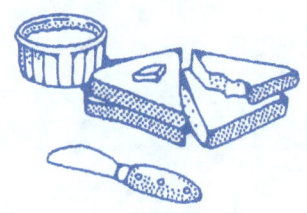 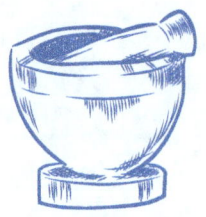

Ingredients:

1 cup black tea
½ cup almond milk
1 tbsp vanilla protein powder
½ cup plain yogurt
1 banana, sliced
1 cup blueberry
2 cups ice
sliced almond, for serving
approx 14 mg purine

Instructions:

Add the black tea, almond milk, protein powder, yogurt, banana, blueberries, and ice to a blender. Blend until smooth.
Serve in a glass-topped with sliced almonds.

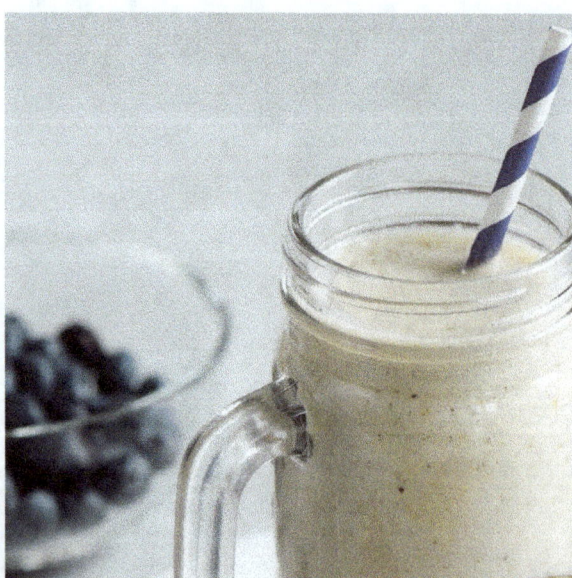

Servings: 4

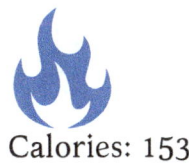
Calories: 153

Ready in 15min

PERSIMMON LASSI

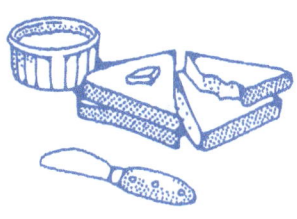

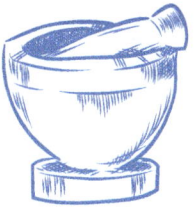

Ingredients:

3 persimmons
1 organic lime
2 cups plain yogurt (1.5 % fat)
2 tsp powdered cardamom
1 tsp honey
6 ice cubes
approx 8 mg purine

Instructions:

Clean, wash, and cut the persimmons into quarters. The lime should be washed, dried, and the peel removed. In a blender, combine the persimmon, honey, lime zest, yogurt, cardamom, and ice cubes and blend on high until a smooth consistency. If possible, add a splash of cold water or lime juice. Serve cold, divided among four glasses.

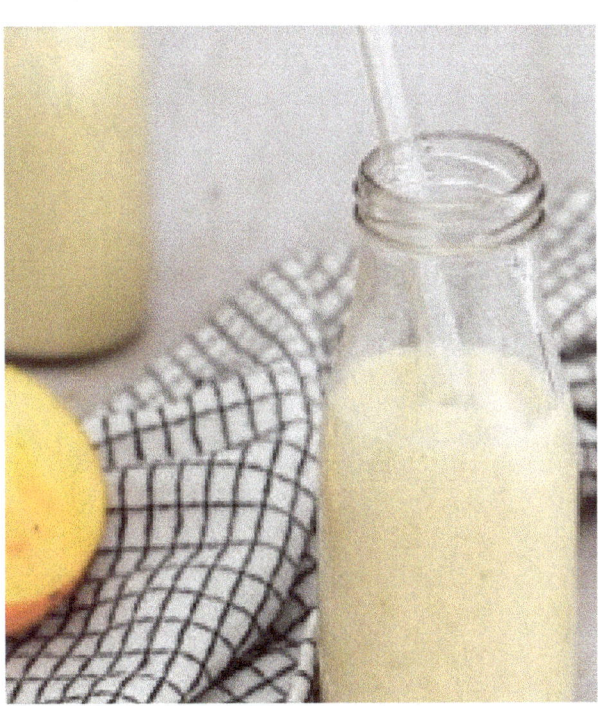

 Servings: 2

 Calories: 495

 Ready in 5 min

COFFEE SMOOTHIE

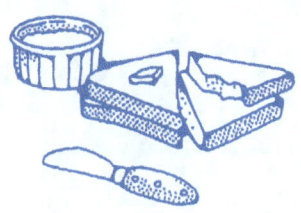

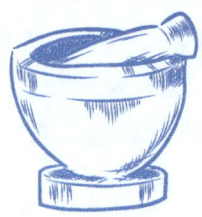

Ingredients:

2 frozen bananas
Coconut water 1 cup
cocoa powder 2 tbsp
4 tbsp espresso coffee
approx 11 mg purine

Instructions:

Combine all ingredients in a blender and puree until smooth. Pour into two glasses and serve chilled.

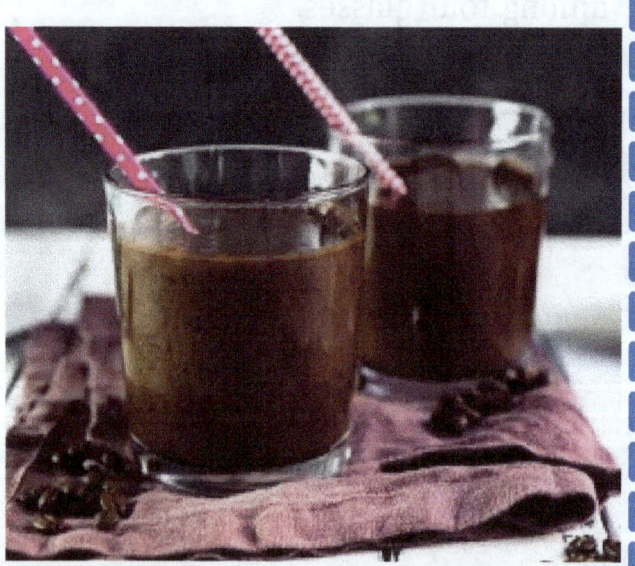

 Servings: 1
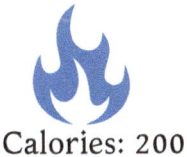 Calories: 200
 Ready in 5 min

CHERRY "CHEESECAKE" SMOOTHIE

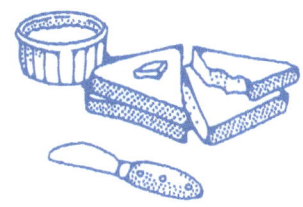
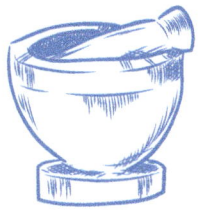

Ingredients:

1 ¼ cup unsweetened coconut milk
¾ cup cherries, frozen
1 tbsp of coconut oil
1 tsp lemon juice (optional)
2 tsp extract de vanille
1 tsp raw honey or pure maple syrup
1 tbsp protein powder (unflavored)
approx 8 mg purine

Instructions:

In a high-powered blender, mix the cashews and coconut milk until smooth (1-2 minutes).
Mix for another minute on high with the remaining ingredients.
Add ¼ cup more water or coconut milk if the smoothie is too thick for you.

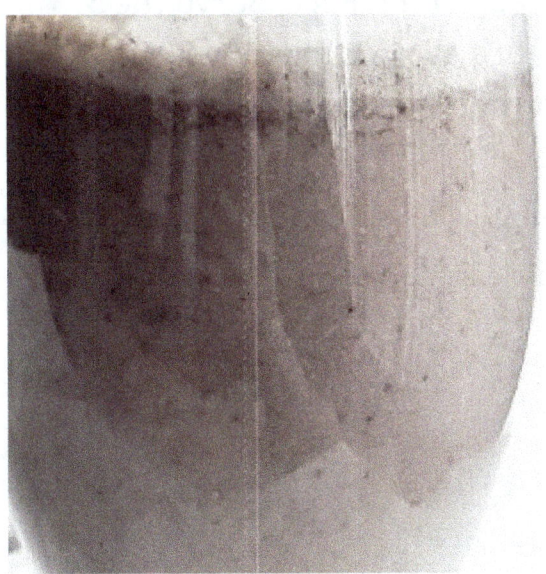

 Servings: 25

 Calories: 33

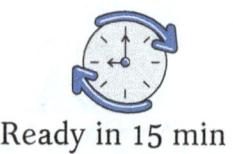 Ready in 15 min

HEALTHY GREEN SHOT

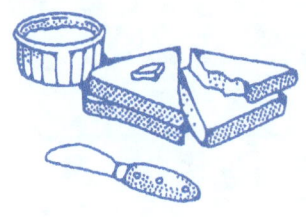

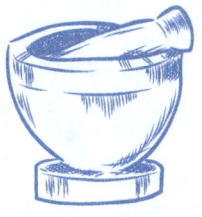

Ingredients:

2 pears
3 green apples (e.g., granny smith)
3 stalk Celery
4 tbsp Ginger (organic)
1 bunch parsley
3 kilograms of kiwifruit
2 Lime
Turmeric, 1 tsp
approx 18 mg purine

Instructions:

Peel, wash, and cut pears, apples, celery, ginger, and parsley. Using a spoon, scrape the pulp from the kiwi fruit halves. Limes should be halved, and the juice squeezed out.
In a blender mix pears, apples, kiwis, celery, ginger, and parsley.
Season with turmeric and freshly squeezed lime juice. Serve the mixture as shots right away or portion it out and freeze it.

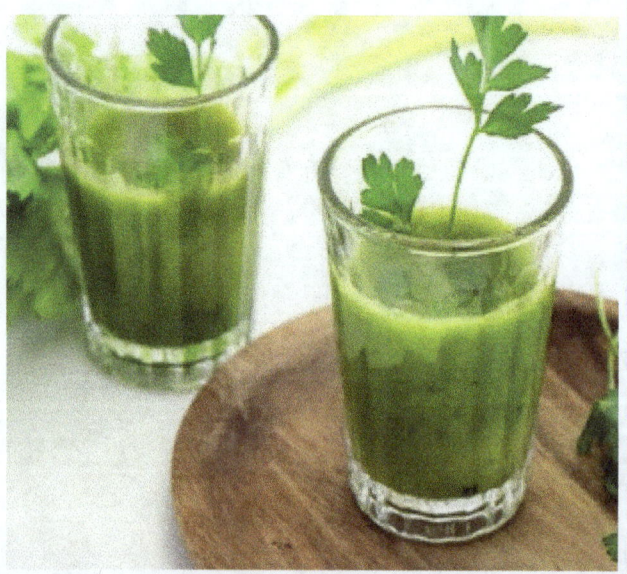

Servings: 3

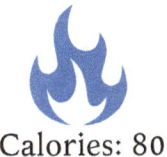
Calories: 80

Ready in 5min

CHERRY CHOCOLATE SMOOTHIE

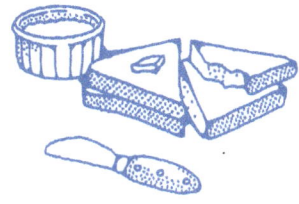

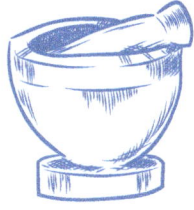

Ingredients:

8 ounces coconut water
2 cups fresh or frozen pitted cherries
1 ice cube
2 tbsp cocoa powder (unsweetened)
optional garnish: chopped cherries
approx 9 mg purine

Instructions:

Place cherries, coconut water, ice, and unsweetened cocoa powder in a blender and blend until smooth. As an optional garnish, top with sliced fresh cherries.

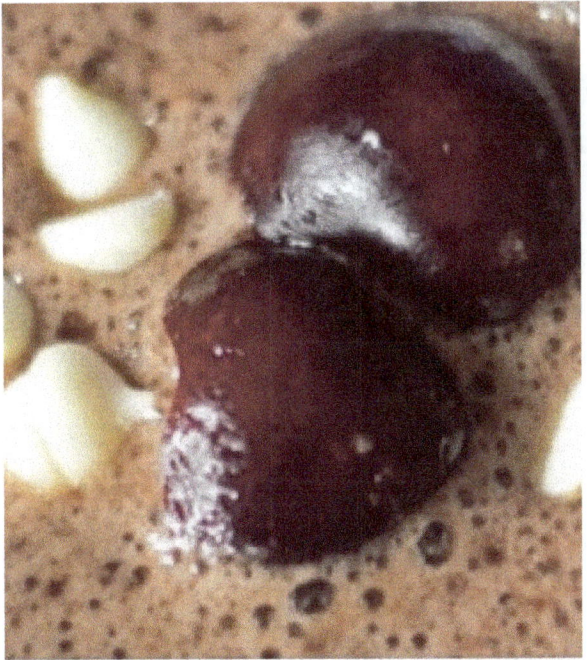

 Servings: 2   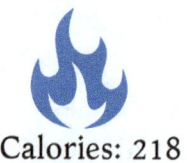 Calories: 218    Ready in 10min

MANGO AND BANANA SMOOTHIE

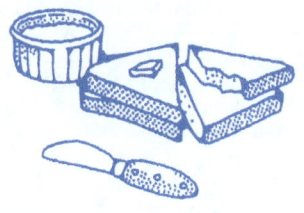 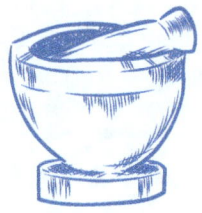

Ingredients:

1 small ripe mango
5 oranges
1 banana,
1 cup Yogurt (low-fat)
approx 18 mg purine

Instructions:

Squeeze the oranges to get the juice. Blend a banana, mango after removing the skin, yogurt, and orange juice until smooth.
Serve in two glasses.

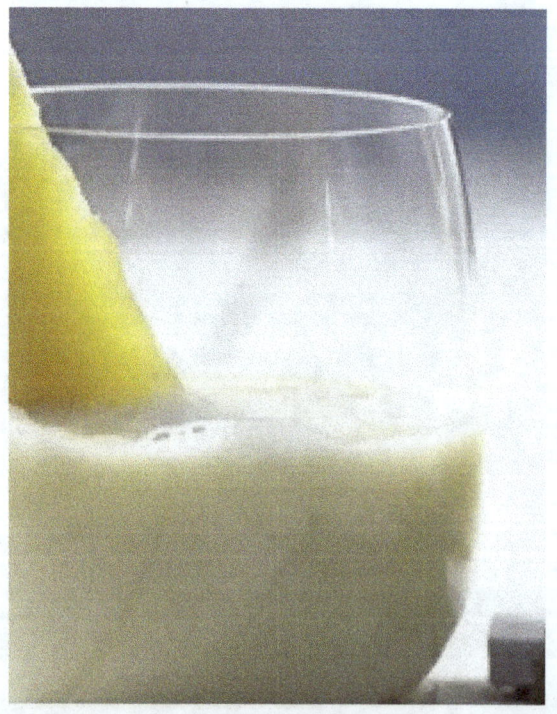

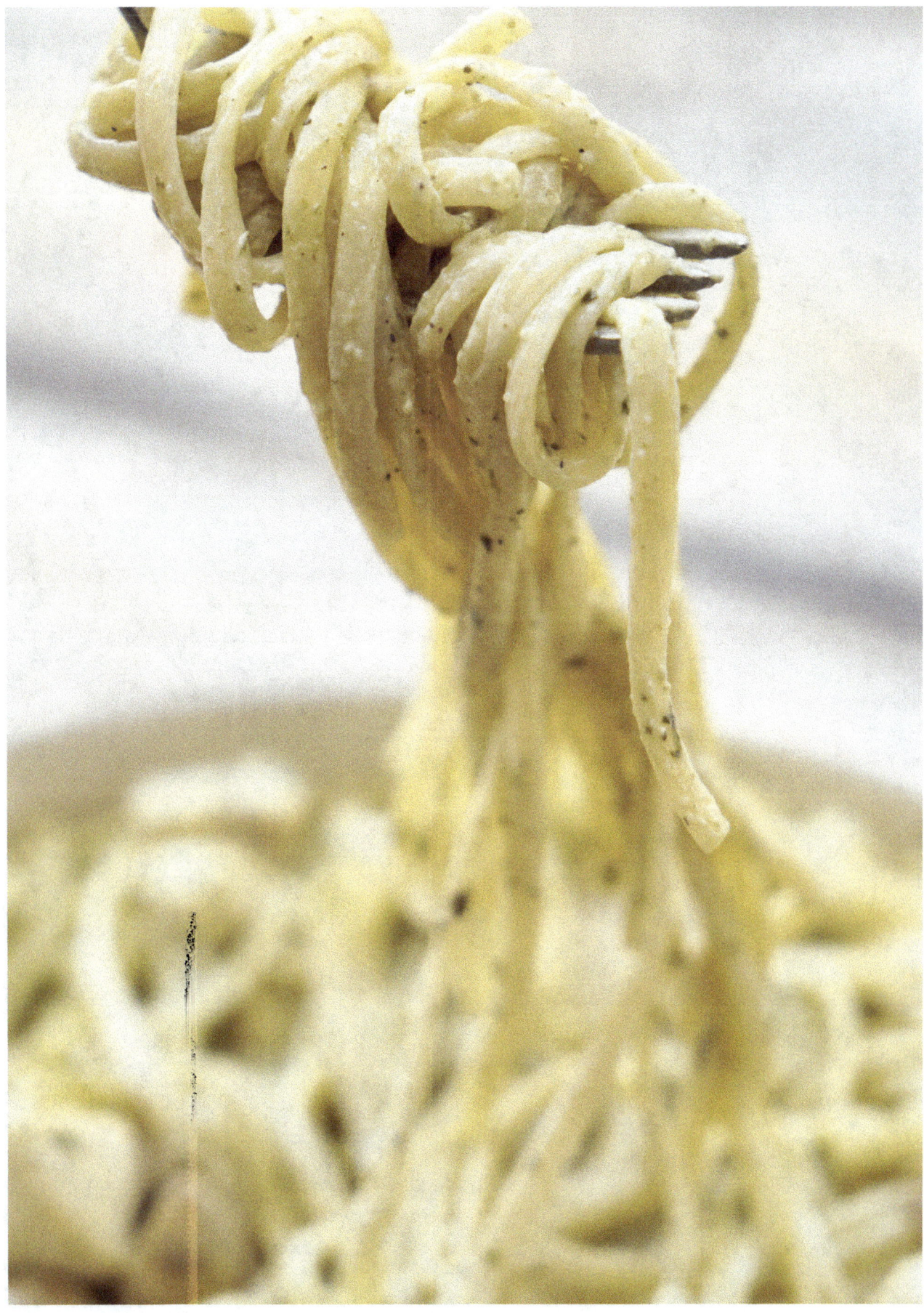

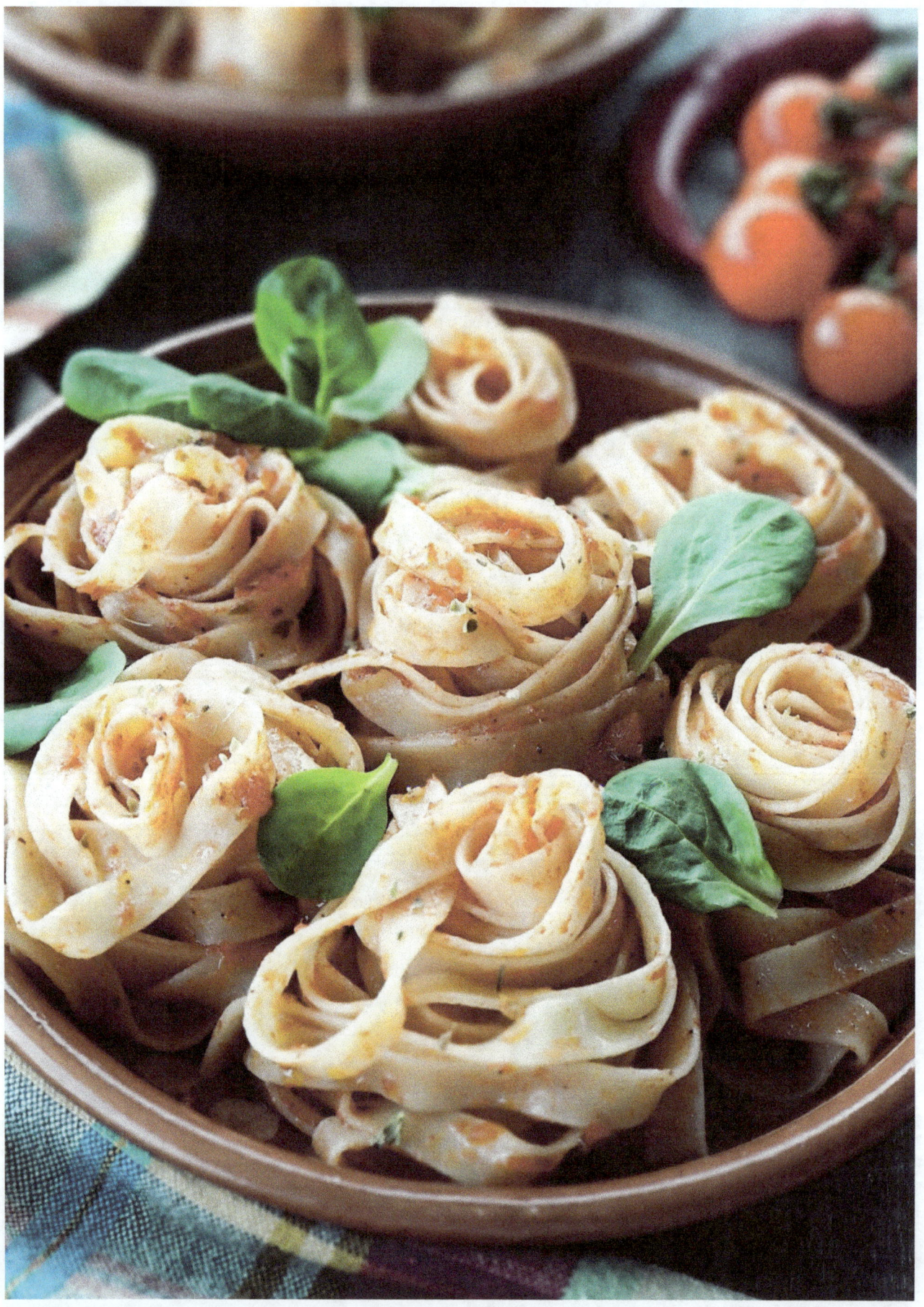

PASTA

RICE

 Servings: 4

 Calories: 386

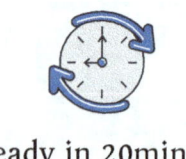 Ready in 20min

ZUCCHINI SPAGHETTI

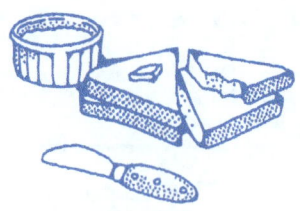

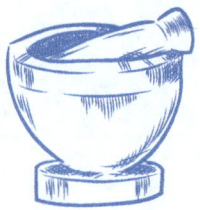

Ingredients:

1 (7-ounce) can of chipotle chiles in adobo sauce
1 hot chili
2 cups spaghetti
2 tbsp olive oil
2 minced garlic cloves
4 cups shredded zucchini
a quarter tsp of salt
a quarter tsp of black pepper
2 tbsp grated Parmesan cheese
approx 32 mg purine

Instructions:

Cook pasta as directed on the box. Remove the seeds from the chili (leave the seeds in for extra heat); mince the chile. In a wide nonstick skillet, heat the oil over medium-high heat. Sauté for 1 minute with the chili, sauce, and garlic. Add the zucchini and cook for 4 minutes, stirring continuously. Combine pasta and zucchini mixture in a large mixing bowl—season with salt, pepper, and parmesan cheese.

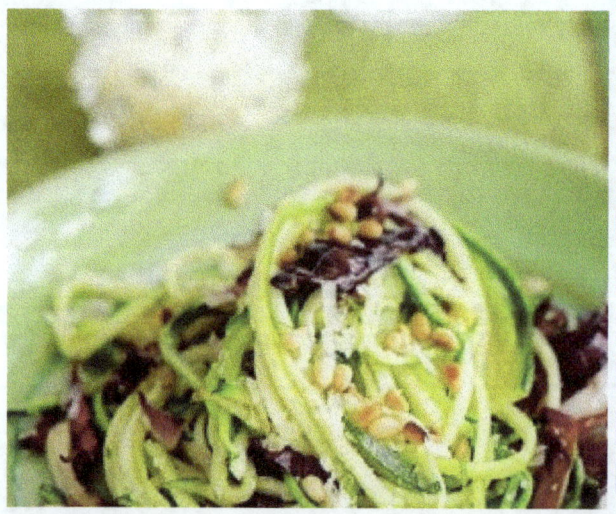

 Servings: 4    Calories: 531    Ready in 30 min

LENTIL NOODLES WITH PESTO

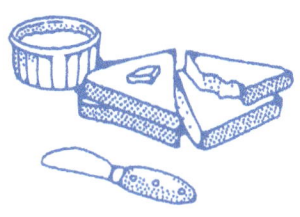

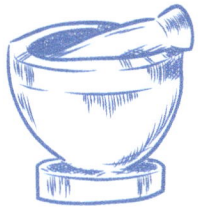

Ingredients:

2 cups brussels sprouts
1 cup lentil noodles
1 garlic clove
5 tbsp oil-dried tomato (drained)
parmesan cheese in a single piece
2 tbsp Pinenuts
8 tbsp olive oil
2 lemons (organic) (zest and juice)
cayenne pepper
1 handful basil leaves
approx 48 mg purine

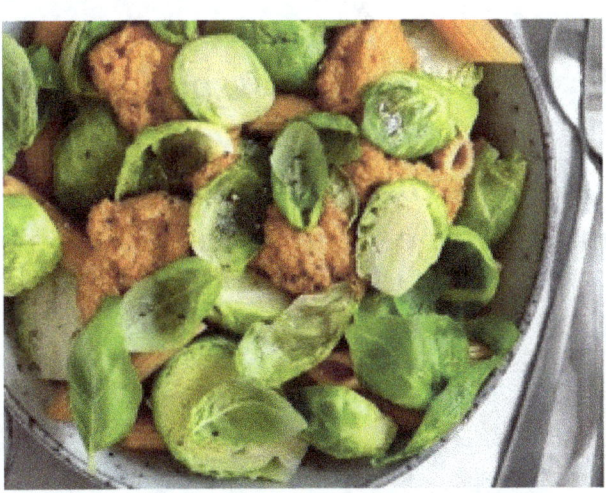

Instructions:

Thoroughly clean, wash, and cut the Brussels sprouts in half. Boil the sprouts for 5 minutes in salted water. Drain and rinse.
Meanwhile, boil the pasta as directed on the package.
Cut the dried tomatoes into small pieces in the meantime. Parmesan cheese should be grated and roast pinenuts in a hot pan without fat over medium heat.
Using a blender, finely puree the tomatoes, parmesan, pinenuts, oil, and 3–4 tbsps water. Season to taste with salt, pepper, lemon zest, and juice. Clean the basil by squeezing it dry. Serve with pesto and basil on top of the pasta and Brussels sprouts.

Servings: 1

Calories: 590

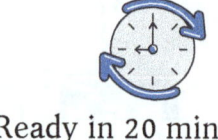
Ready in 20 min

GOAT CHEESE PASTA

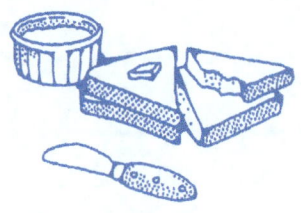
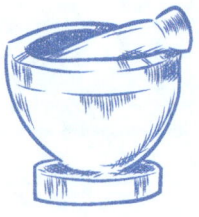

Ingredients:

1 small garlic clove
2 dry tomatoes in oil
3 basil stems
60 g goat cheese
80 g pasta (whole wheat) (e.g., linguine)
cumin
approx 30 mg purine

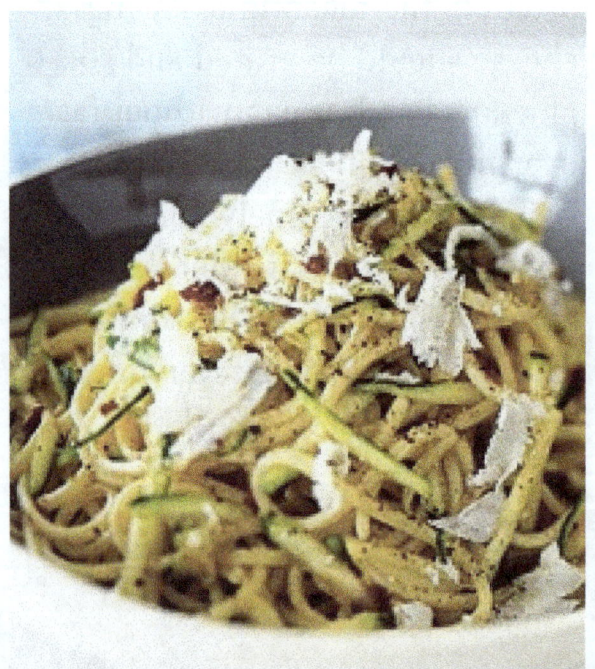

Instructions:

Place the tomatoes in a colander and pour the oil into a small cup. Cut the tomatoes into strips or roughly slice them with a sharp knife. Peel and finely cut the garlic cloves. Wash the basil leaves, shake them out, and cut them coarsely. Through your fingers, break up the goat cheese. Cook the noodles until they are firm to the bite in plenty of salted water according to the package directions. Meanwhile, heat tomato oil in a pan over low heat fry garlic and tomatoes for a few minutes in the oil. Combine the basil and goat cheese in a bowl and stir to combine. Drain the pasta, mix in the goat cheese pasta, add fry tomatoes and garlic, and season with black pepper.

 Servings: 2

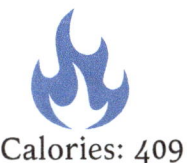 Calories: 409

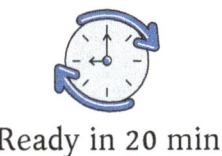 Ready in 20 min

KONJAC PASTA WITH BERRIES

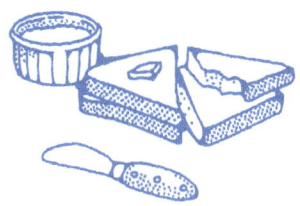

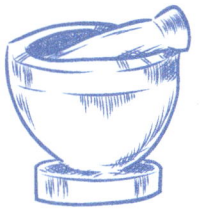

Ingredients:

1 lime
2 shallots
1 garlic clove
1 chili pepper (red)
3 sticks celery
rapeseed oil, 2 tbsp
Vegetable broth ½ cup
1 cup soy cream or almond cuisine
2 tbsp Pine nuts
5 big strawberries
half bunch parsley
cayenne pepper
2 cups konjac noodles
approx 28 mg purine

Instructions:

Wash the lime in hot water, pat dry, and grate some peel finely. Squeeze the juice from Lime.

Peel shallots and garlic and finely dice them. Cut the chili half lengthwise, core it, wash it, and chop it. Celery should be cleaned, threads removed if possible, washed, and cut into thick slices. Chop the celery greens coarsely.

In a pan, heat the oil. Sauté for 3–4 minutes over medium heat with shallots, garlic, chili, and celery. Use broth to deglaze the pan. Pour in the almond or soy cream, bring to a boil, and cook for 5–6 minutes, stirring occasionally.

Meanwhile, toast the pine nuts for 3 minutes in a hot pan without fat over medium heat. Strawberries should be cleaned and washed before being cut into small cubes. Parsley should be washed, dried, and chopped.

Add the parsley into the sauce and mix well—season with salt, pepper, lime zest, and juice to taste. Boil konjak spaghetti for 2 minutes in salted boiling water. Drain and combine with the herb and lime sauce. Serve on a plate of pine nuts and strawberries on top.

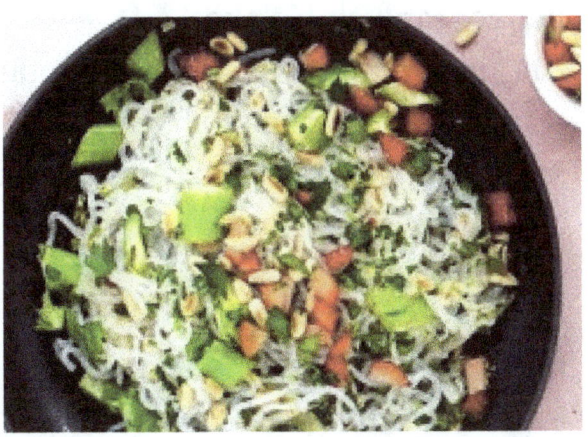

 Servings: 2

 Calories: 542

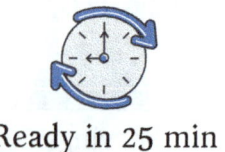 Ready in 25 min

SPAGHETTI WITH PAK CHOI

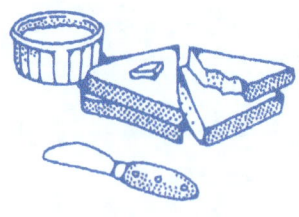

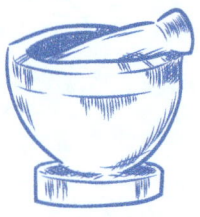

Ingredients:

1 cup whole wheat spaghetti
2 tbsp ginger
1 clove of garlic
2 pieces spring onions
2 cups pak choi
1 handful parsley
1 tbsp coconut oil
1 tbsp lime juice
pepper
chili flakes
1 tsp sesame
approx 28 mg purine

Instructions:

Boil the spaghetti in salted boiling water for about 8-10 minutes until al dente. Then drain.

In the meantime, peel and chop the ginger and garlic. Clean and wash the spring onions and cut them into rings. Clean and wash the pak choi and cut it into strips. Wash the parsley and shake dry.

Heat the oil in a pan, sauté the ginger, garlic, and spring onions over medium heat for 4 minutes. Add pak choi and sauté for 5 minutes, deglaze with lime juice—season with salt, pepper, and chili flakes.

Arrange the noodles on plates, pour the pak choi on top and serve sprinkled with parsley, sesame seeds, and chili flakes

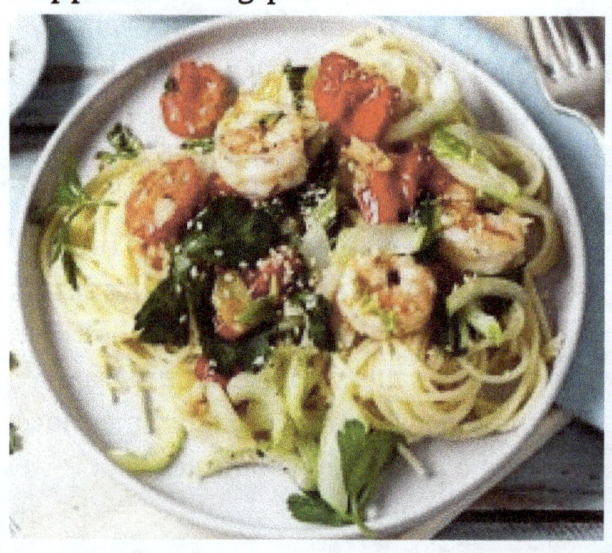

Servings: 2

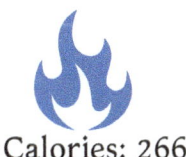
Calories: 266

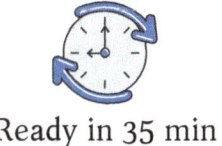
Ready in 35 min

ZUCCHINI PASTA

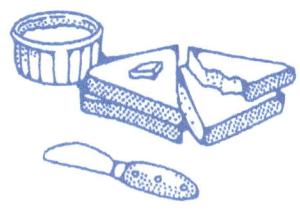

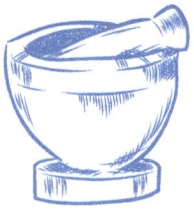

Ingredients:

2 tbsp pine nuts
2 radicchio
2 cups zucchini
1 clove of garlic
1 tbsp olive oil
1 organic lemon
1 tbsp walnut oil
pepper
approx 18 mg purine

Instructions:

Roast the pine nuts in a large pan until they are fragrant. Take out and let cool. Wash the radicchio and cut it into strips.

Wash and clean the zucchini. Use a spiral cutter to cut into fine linguine strips. Peel garlic and chop finely. Wash the lemon with hot water and pat dry. Finely grate the peel and squeeze out the juice.

Heat the pine nut pan again and add the olive oil. Add the garlic, radicchio, and sauté for 1–2 minutes over low heat.

Then remove from heat and add zucchini, lemon juice, lemon zest, and walnut oil. Season with salt and pepper and season to taste. Divide between 2 plates and sprinkle with pine nuts.

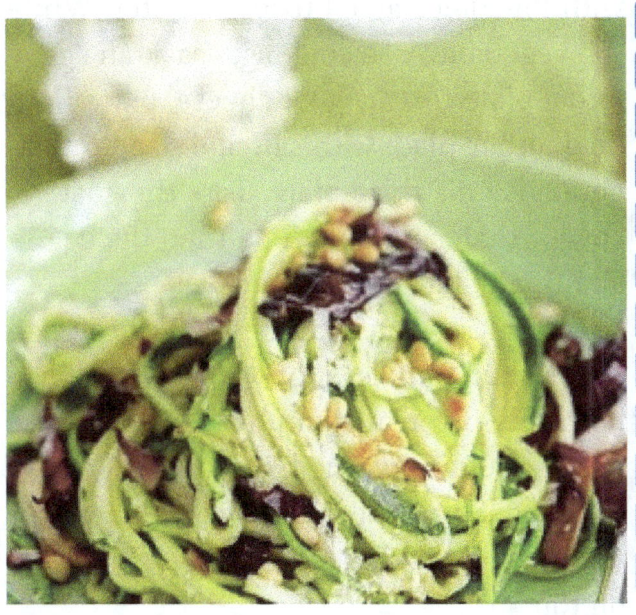

Servings: 2

Calories: 629

Ready in 30min

GOAT CHEESE RICE PAN

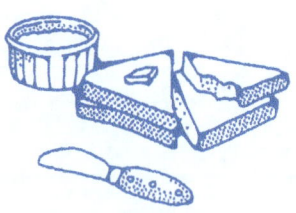

Ingredients:
1 cup parboiled rice
1 tsp salt
2 tbsp turmeric powder
1 shallot
1 garlic clove
2 carrots
1 pepper, red
1 lime, organic
2 tbsps olive oil
cayenne pepper
4 thaler of goat cheese
1 ice cube
2 tbsp spelled wholemeal flour
3 tbsp almond flour
a quarter-bunch of basil
oil for fry
approx 20 mg purine

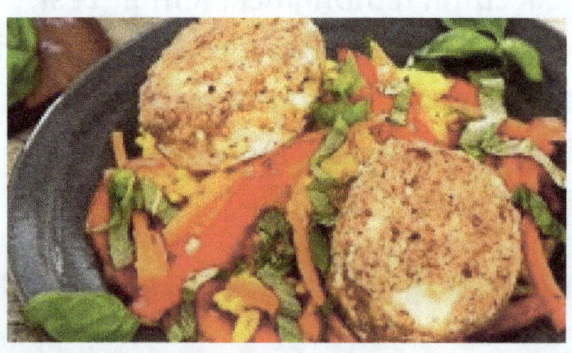

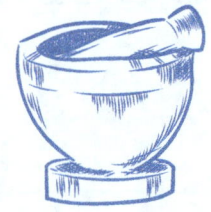

Instructions:
Boil rice for 16-18 minutes over low heat in 1 cup boiling salted water with turmeric. Then remove it from the heat and set it aside to steep.
Peel and cut the shallot and garlic in the meantime. Carrots and peppers should be cleaned and washed before being cut into strips. Rinse the lime in hot water, dry it, rub the peel, and squeeze the juice into a glass. In a pan, heat 1 tbsp of oil, and over medium heat, sauté the shallot and garlic for 2 minutes. Sauté for 5-7 minutes with the carrot and bell pepper strips. Cook for 2 minutes after adding the rice. Season with salt, pepper, deglazing the rice pan with lime juice and 3 tbsps of water. While the vegetables are cooking, crack an egg into a plate for the goat cheese, place flour on another plate with salt and pepper and almonds on a third plate. Toss the goat cheese thaler in flour first, then the egg, and finally into the almonds.
In a separate pan, heat the oil. Fry the goat's cheese thalers for 7-8 minutes on both sides over medium heat, until golden. Basil should be washed, dried, and chopped. Serve the goat cheese thaler alongside the rice pan and a sprig of basil on top.

 Servings: 2

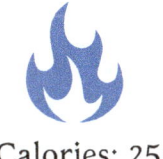 Calories: 250

 Ready in 25 min

COUSCOUS BASE RECIPE

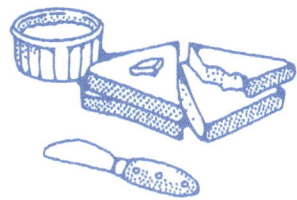

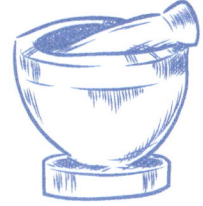

Ingredients:

1 cup cuscus,
1 cup water,
salt,
olive oil
approx 0 mg purine

Instructions:

Fry cuscus in a pan with olive oil stir all the time with a wooden spoon until it changes the color; put the cuscus in a bowl through over salted boiling water and cover. You can boil in the water Rosmarin or thyme or some aromatic leaves if you want to. Wait for around 15 min so the couscous will absorb all water and double the volume.

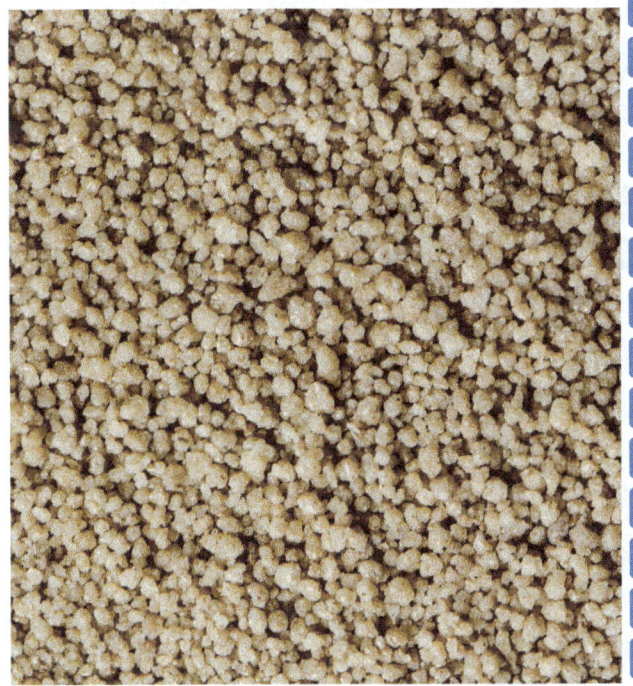

 Servings: 2

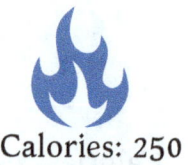 Calories: 250

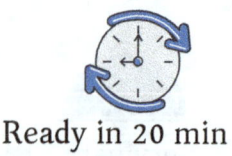 Ready in 20 min

COUSCOUS WITH VEGETABLES

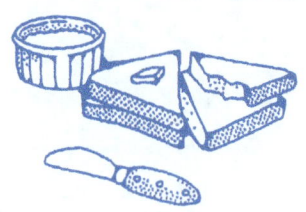

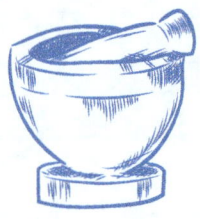

Ingredients:

1 cup cuscus
1 cups water
2 onions,
3 carrots,
2 courgettes
2 garlic cloves,
rosemary,
olive oil,
salt
approx 12 mg purine

Instructions:

Wash and cut long way carrots and courgettes. Cut the onion and fry them in a pan with oil until soft, add carrots, and after 5 min, add courgettes.
In the end, add finely cut garlic, rosemary, and salt, cover the pan and let on medium heat for 15 minutes.
Make ready cuscus as in the base recipe. Stir cuscus with vegetables and serve.

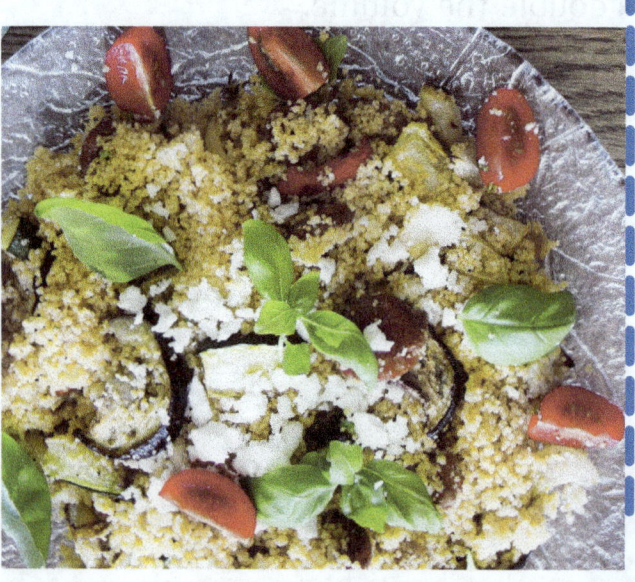

 Servings: 4

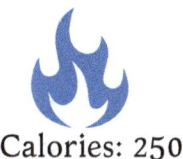 Calories: 250

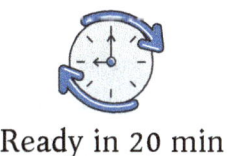 Ready in 20 min

COUSCOUS WITH ROSEMARY

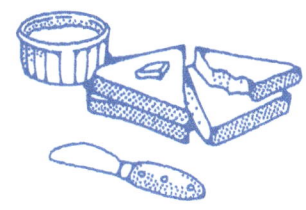

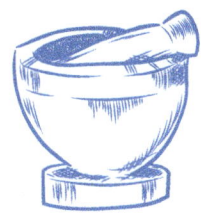

Ingredients:

1 cup cuscus
1 cups water
2 tablespoons of soy sauce (if you wish to)
rosemary
olive oil
salt
approx 0 mg purine

Instructions:

Toasty cuscus with oil and rosemary, as described in the base recipe.
Boil water with soy sauce. Put the cuscus in the bowl through boil water on and cover. Leave for 15 min. Serve on a plate, ideally with vegetables.

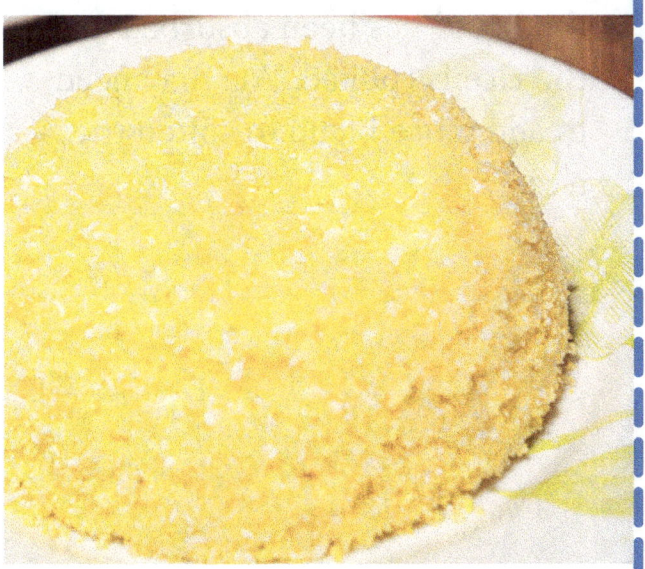

Servings: 8

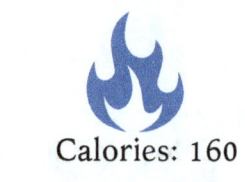
Calories: 160

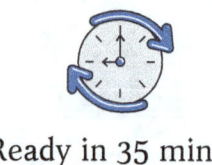
Ready in 35 min

EASY RICE

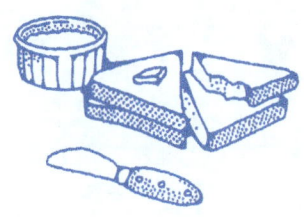
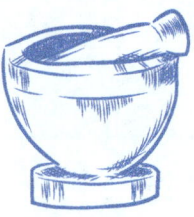

Ingredients:

1 cup kidney beans / red peas
2 sprigs of fresh thyme
1 bay leaf
1 spring onion
1 tsp cumin powder
1 clove garlic finely chopped
½ tsp all-purpose seasoning
1 red pepper deseeded and diced
½ cup frozen mixed vegetables
1 cup basmati rice uncooked
4 tbsp coconut cream
2 cups water
approx 86 mg purine

Instructions:

Put the beans in a large pan with a tight-fitting lid and add the water. Then add all the other ingredients, except the rice, and bring to a boil. Rinse the rice in warm water before adding it to the pot. Stir well.

Cover the pan and simmer for a further 20-30 minutes or until all the liquid has been absorbed and the rice is cooked. You may need to add more liquid to soften the rice.

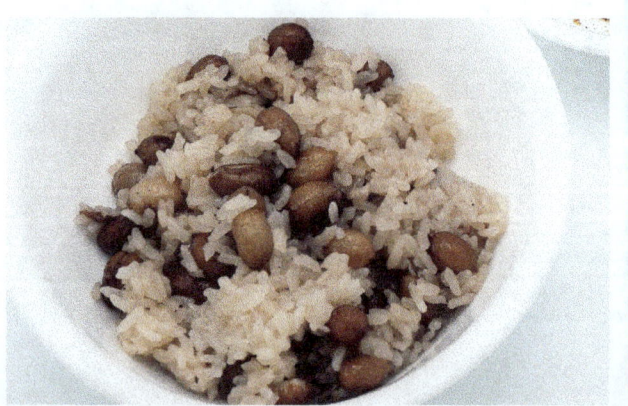

Servings: 4

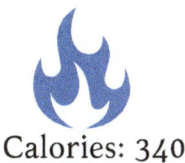
Calories: 340

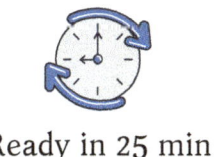
Ready in 25 min

PASTA WITH EGGS

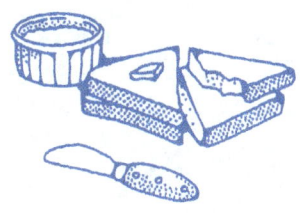

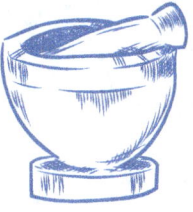

Ingredients:

2 cups pasta
6 small courgettes,
1 onion,
half red pepper
1 leaf carbage,
2 eggs,
nutmeg,
Parmigiano Reggiano cheese,
olive oil, salt
approx 20 mg purine

Instructions:

Wash and cut on small pieces the vegetable, fry them in the oil, start with onion, pepper, cabbage leaf, and courgette; after adding salt, cover and let them fry on medium heat for 15 min.

In the meantime, boil pasta in a big pot with salted water. In one bowl, whisk eggs with nutmeg. After the pasta is boiled, drain and mix the pasta in the pan with vegetables, add a few spoons of olive oil and eggs and let them mix well for 2 minutes on medium heat. Serve with parmigiano reggiano grated chees on top.

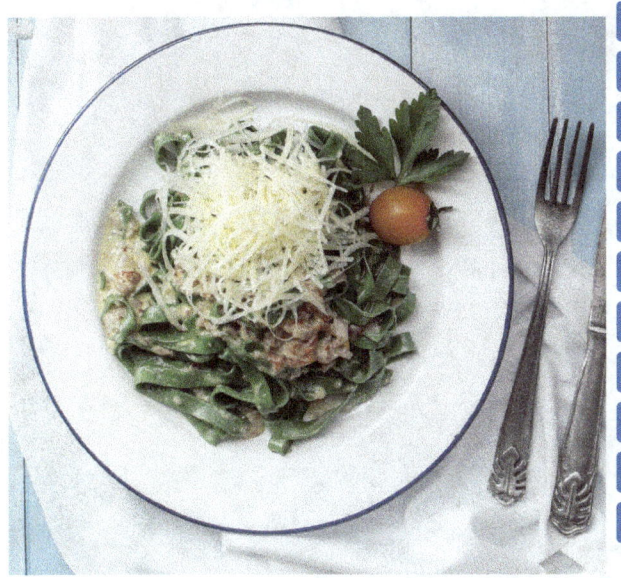

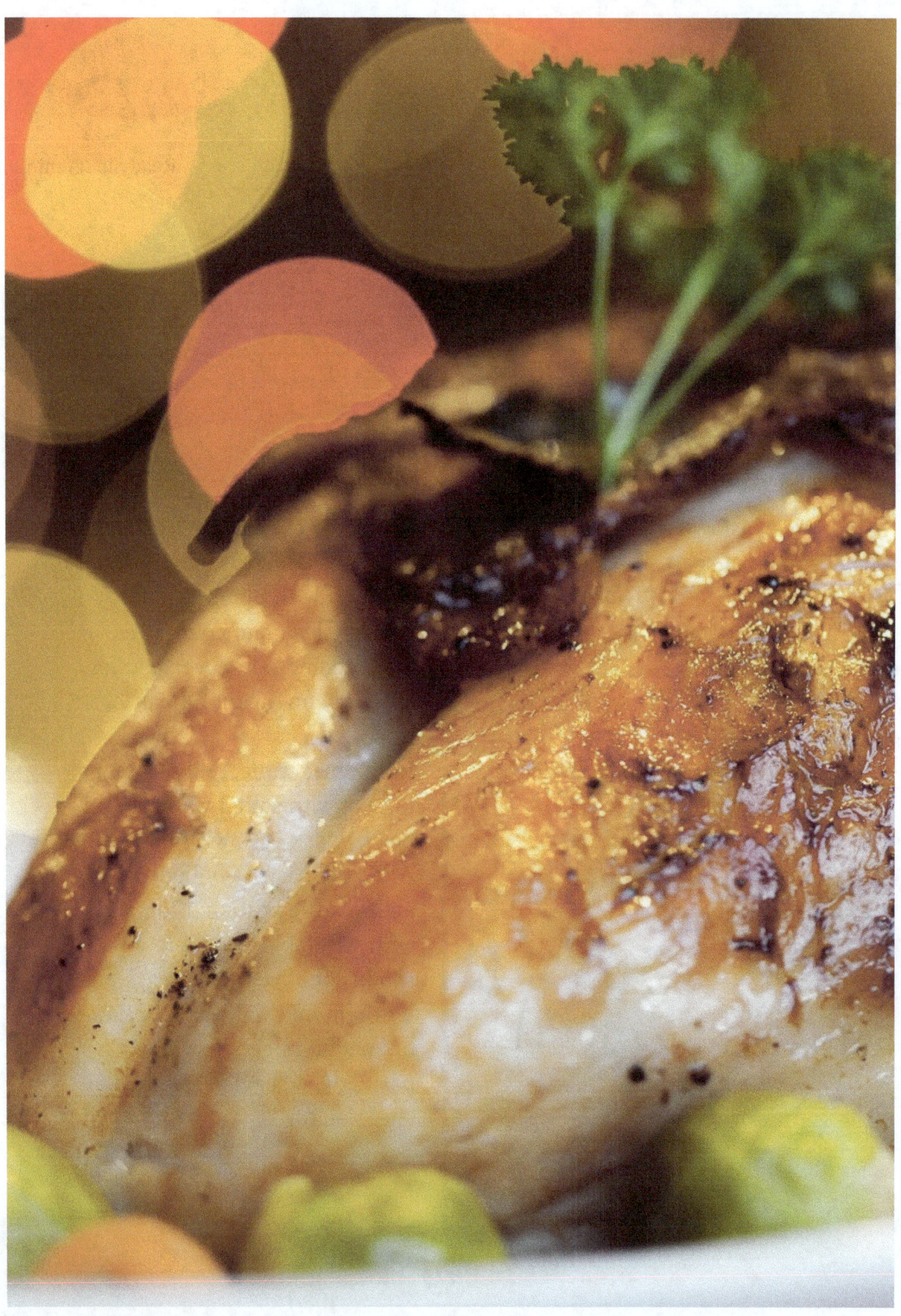

CHICKEN

 Servings: 4  Calories: 357 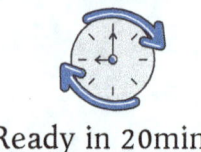 Ready in 20min

CHICKEN AND VEGETABLE FRIED RICE

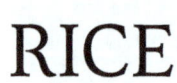

Ingredients:

1 cup diced chicken breast
1 medium onion, diced
1 medium diced zucchini
Cut 1 ear of corn kernels
1 cup peas (green)
½ cup shelled and cooked edamame
2 cups cooked broccoli, cut into small florets
1 egg
2 cups brown rice leftovers, ideally cold
1 tbsp sesame oil
2 tbsp low-sodium soy sauce
1 tbsp of vinegar
1 cup minced scallions
approx 150 mg purine

Instructions:

Spray a wok or wide pan with non-stick spray and heat over medium-high heat. Cook chicken breasts for 4 minutes on each side. There's no need to keep moving the chicken around; let it brown and flavor.

When the chicken is finished, remove it from the pan and set it aside.

Cook for 3-4 minutes in the same pan the onion and zucchini.

Combine corn kernels, peas, edamame, and broccoli in a frying pan, and fry for 2 minutes

Arrange the vegetables around the pan's edge, then crack the egg in the middle. Scramble the egg with a wooden spoon as soon as possible.

Combine the cold brown rice, cooked chicken, and sesame oil. Stir well to disperse the oil and evenly distribute the rice and vegetables in the pan.

Allow the ingredients to brown slightly for 3 min. approx. Mix in the scallions, soy sauce, and rice vinegar.

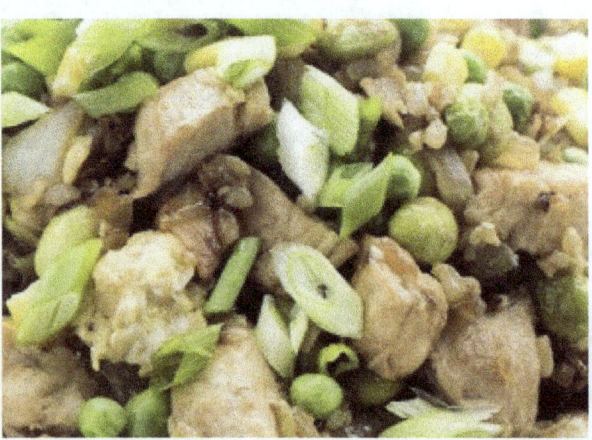

 Servings: 4

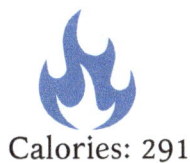 Calories: 291

 Ready in 30 min

CHICKEN SALAD

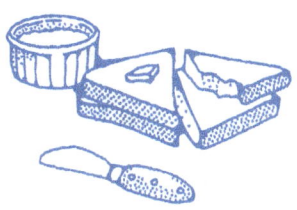

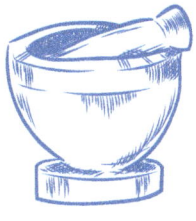

Ingredients:

2 boneless, skinless chicken breasts, cooked and cut into cubes
2 celery stalks, chopped
1 tbsp red onion, chopped
1/2 cup quartered red seedless grapes
1/2 cup non-fat Greek yogurt
1 tsp powdered garlic
1 tsp freshly ground black pepper
2 halved whole-wheat pita pockets
4 lettuce leaves
approx 70 mg purine

Instructions:

Add all of the salad ingredients together in a big mixing bowl. Mix well. You can eat the chicken salad on its own or in a pita sandwich.

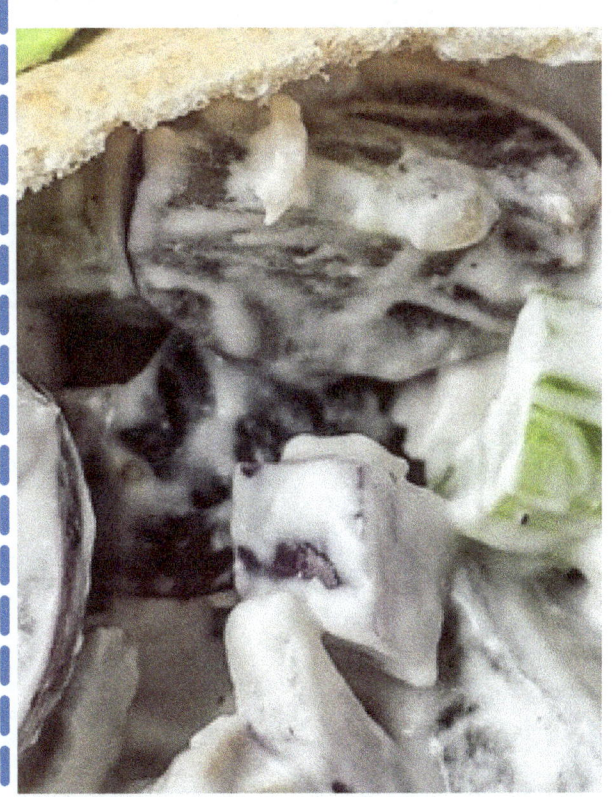

 Servings: 8    Calories: 180    Ready 1hour

BROWN STEW CHICKEN

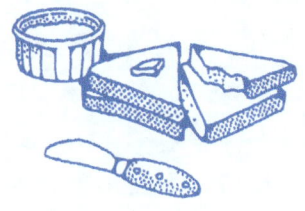

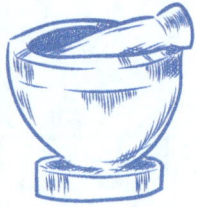

Ingredients:

6 chicken quarters - skin removed
1 carrot peeled and diced
1 green or red pepper finely sliced
1 cup water

Marinade
1 tsp coarsely ground black pepper
3 sprigs thyme
1 tbsp low sodium soy sauce
1 clove of garlic crushed
1 large tomato chopped
1 medium onion chopped
juice of 1 lime
scotch bonnet pepper to taste
approx 180 mg purine

Instructions:

Coat the chicken with garlic, soy sauce, onion, black pepper, lime juice, and scotch bonnet pepper. Marinate in the fridge for about 2 hours or overnight, if possible.

Preheat the oven to 190 C / 370 F. Meanwhile, mix all the other ingredients and water in the chicken marinade.

Cover with foil or a tight-fitting lid and bake in the oven for 30-40 minutes, turning frequently.

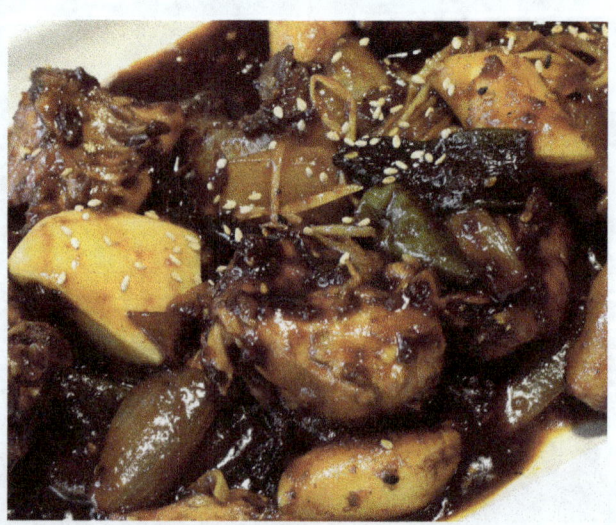

 Servings: 4
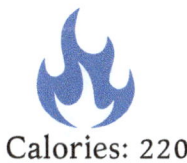 Calories: 220
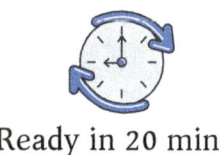 Ready in 20 min

CHICKEN VEGGIE

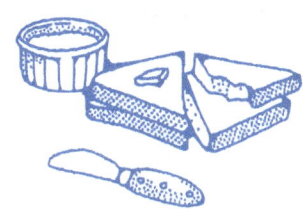

Ingredients:

2 tbsp low-sodium soy sauce, divided
1 lime juice, split
2 tbsp sesame oil (divided)
2 cups chicken breast, skinless and boneless, cut into bite-size parts
1 tbsp canola oil, expeller pressed
2 carrots, peeled and sliced into tiny rounds (about 1 cup)
2 cups broccoli florets, cut into bite-size pieces (from 1 small bunch)
1 medium zucchini, sliced lengthwise in half and then into 14-inch-thick half-moons (about 2 cups)
4 minced garlic cloves
2 green onions (white and green parts)
1 seeded and minced jalapeno pepper
¼ cup new basil, sliced
¼ cup fresh cilantro, chopped
Brown rice, if desired
approx 180 mg purine

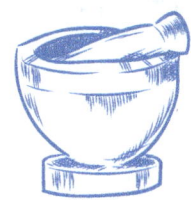

Instructions:

In a big zip-top plastic bag or cup, combine 1 tbsp soy sauce, ginger, half a lime juice, and 1 tsp sesame oil. Place the chicken pieces in the zip-top plastic bag or cup, mix them all well, and place them in the refrigerator for 1 hour or up to 24 hours.

Heat the oil in a large wok or non-stick skillet over medium-high heat when you're ready to make your stir fry.

Stir in the chicken and the marinade for 1 minute. Stir in the carrots, broccoli, zucchini, garlic, green onions, and jalapeno pepper for a few minutes more, or until the chicken is cooked through and the vegetables are crisp-tender.

Combine the remaining 1 tbsp soy sauce, the remaining lime juice, and the remaining sesame oil in a large mixing bowl. Stir in the basil and cilantro just before serving.

If needed, serve with brown rice.

 Servings: 2  Calories: 249  Ready in 45 min

CHICKEN-BROCCOLI STIR FRY

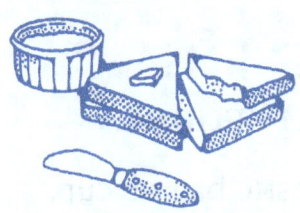
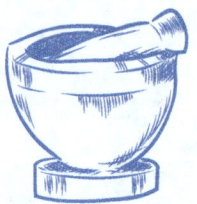

Ingredients:

1 cup low-sodium vegetable broth
1 tbsp low sodium soy sauce
1/2 tsp sesame seed, roasted
White pepper, 1/4 tsp
1/4 to 1/3 tsp thickening
2 cups boneless and skinless chicken thighs or breasts
2 cups blanched broccoli
1/3 cup sliced bell pepper
1/3 cup sliced onion
1 tbsp. minced garlic
1 tbsp. minced ginger
1 tsp of peanut oil
approx 200 mg purine

Instructions:

Prepare the broccoli by blanching it: Fill a large pot halfway with water and bring to a boil.
Separate the florets from the broccoli stem and cut the florets into smile pieces.
Keep a big bowl of ice water near the boiling water tank.
Cook the florets for two to three minutes in boiling water.
Remove the broccoli from the boiling water with a slotted spoon and put it in the ice water.
When cooled, pour into a colander to drain.
Prepare the sauce.
To a cup of vegetable broth, add 1 tsp soy sauce, sesame oil, white pepper, and Thick-It-Up.
Be sure to give it a nice stir. Keep the sauce apart.
continue to the next page

 Servings: 2

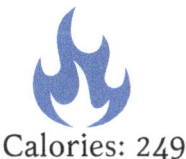 Calories: 249

 Ready in 45min

CHICKEN-BROCCOLI STIR FRY

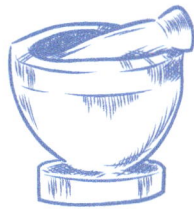

Instructions:

continue from the previous page

In a medium-high-heat pan, combine 1 tbsp peanut oil, 1 tbsp garlic, and 1 tbsp ginger.

Add the onion and bell pepper when the ginger and garlic are fragrant. After a few minutes of stirring, transfer all to the side in the pan.

Place the chicken in the pan's center and spread it out evenly. Allow the chicken to sit for about a minute to develop color on the exterior before flipping it over to build color on the other side. Begin stirring until the exterior of the chicken no longer appears raw.

Turn the heat up to high and stir in the stir fry sauce. Boil, then reduce to low heat and simmer for three minutes, uncovered. Stir in the broccoli and cook until tender.

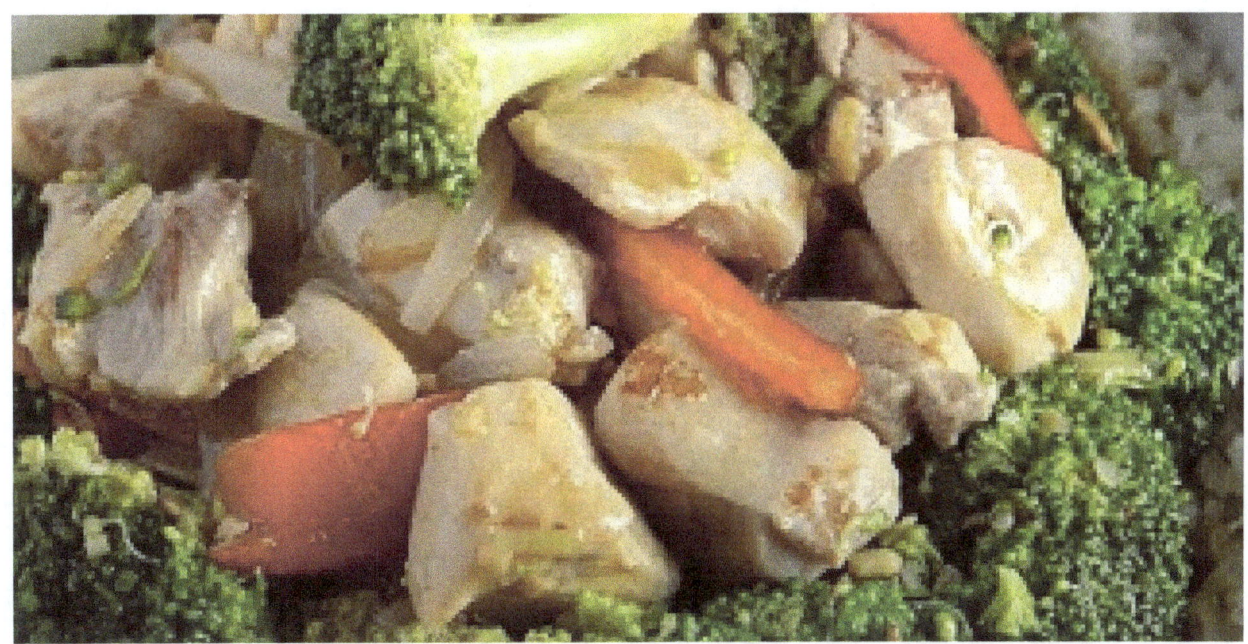

Servings: 4

Calories: 349

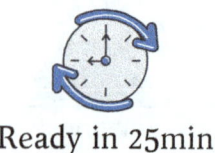
Ready in 25min

CHICKEN WRAP

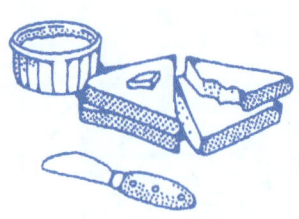

Ingredients:

2 chicken breast fillets
3 tbsp low sodium soy sauce
2 cucumbers
2 carrots
4 coriander stems
8 iceberg lettuce sheets
½ cup of peanut butter
6 tbsps coconut milk
1 tbsp extra virgin olive oil
pepper cayenne
4 tortilla cake (whole grain)
4 tbsp sour cream
approx 75 mg purine

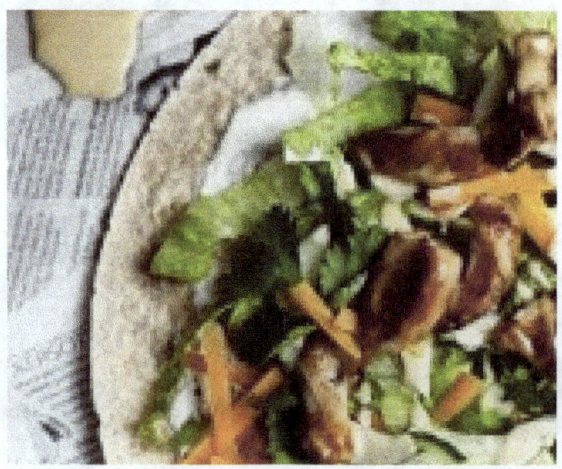

Instructions:

Clean the chicken breasts, dry them, and cut them into strips. In a dish, add 1 tbsp soy sauce, season with salt and pepper, and marinate the chicken breast for about 10 minutes. Meanwhile, wash and cut the cucumber and carrot into fine sticks. Coriander leaves should be cleaned, shaken dry, and loosely chopped. Iceberg lettuce should be washed, dried, and cut into thin strips. Heat the peanut butter and coconut milk together in a saucepan to make the peanut coconut sauce. Season with cayenne pepper and the remaining soy sauce to taste. In a non-stick pan, heat the oil, remove the chicken breast from the marinade, and fry until golden brown on all sides over medium heat. Remove the chicken from the pan and set it aside.

In a non-stick pan, roast wraps for about 30 seconds on each hand. Then, brush one-half of each wrap with 1 tbsp sour cream and top with chicken, cucumber, carrot, and lettuce. Sprinkle coriander and drizzle with peanut and coconut sauce. From the bottom, fold in the chicken wrap and roll it up.

 Servings: 4   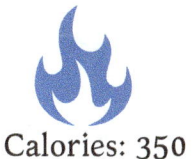 Calories: 350   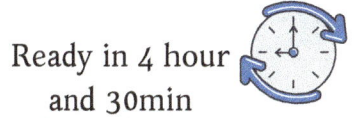 Ready in 4 hour and 30min

CHICKEN WITH GARLIC AND SESAME

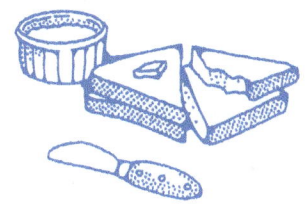   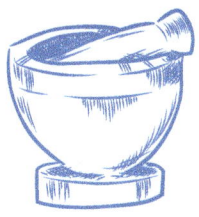

Ingredients:

12 pieces chicken thighs, drumsticks, and legs
4 tbsp water or chicken broth or 1/4 cup tamari coconut aminos may be used as a substitute.
3 garlic cloves, pressed
1 tsp smoked chili pepper (smoked paprika may be substituted)
2 tsp oregano (dried)
2 tbsp apple cider vinegar (unfiltered)
Worcestershire sauce, 2 tsp
1 tbsp sesame oil (toasted)
approx 110 mg purine

Instructions:

Combine all ingredients in a cup, then pour into the slow cooker's bottom. Arrange the chicken on top and pour in the sauce.
Cook for 4 hours on medium.
Serve with your favorite vegetables or rice or quinoa.

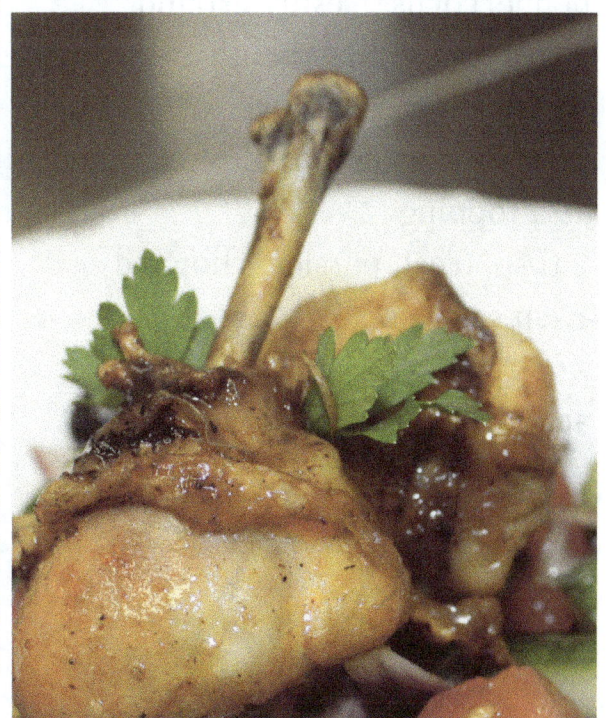

Servings: 4

Calories: 242

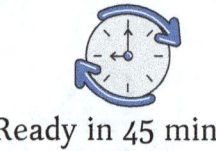
Ready in 45 min

CHICKEN STROGANOFF

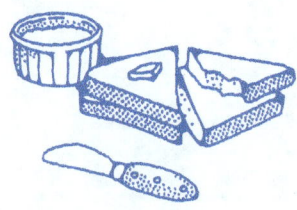

Ingredients:
1 ½ cup wide egg noodles
3 tbsp. unsalted butter
1 small chopped onion
2 cups sliced white or cremini mushrooms
2 cups chicken thighs, skinless and boneless, cut into chunks
2 tbsp flour (all-purpose)
1 tsp paprika, plus additional for sprinkling
peppercorns, freshly ground
1 cup low-sodium broth
1 tbsp Worcestershire
1/2 cup sour cream plus extra to use as a topping
2 tbsp. fresh parsley, chopped
1 tsp salt
¼ tsp pepper
approx 85 mg purine

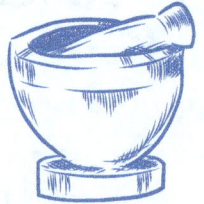

Instructions:
Boil a large pot of salted water, boil the noodles according to the package directions, and drain.

Meanwhile, in a big skillet over medium-high heat, melt 2 tbsp butter, add onion and fry for 2 minutes, or until the onion is slightly soft. Add mushrooms and fry for another 2 minutes.

Mix the chicken, paprika, salt, and pepper with the remaining 1 tbsp butter. Fry, constantly stirring, for 3 minutes, or until the chicken is golden brown.

Add the chicken broth and Worcestershire sauce. Bring to a low boil, reduce to low heat and cook until the sauce has thickened, around 5 minutes. Season with salt and pepper and stir in the sour cream. Boil gently for another 2 minutes, or until the chicken is cooked through. Distribute the noodles between the bowls.

Add the chicken mixture, parsley, sour cream, and paprika to the top.

 Servings: 2 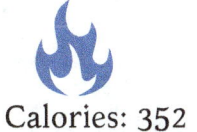 Calories: 352 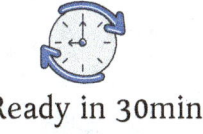 Ready in 30min

LEMON AND ASPARAGUS CHICKEN

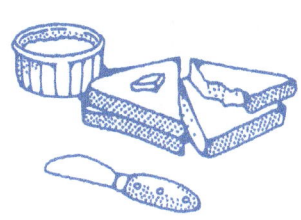

Ingredients:

1 lemon, organic
2 chicken breast fillets
cayenne pepper
powdered paprika
2 tbsp whole wheat flour
2 tbsp olive oil
2 cups asparagus (green)
2 cloves garlic
1 tbsp mustard
½ cup vegetable broth low sodium
a quarter-bunch of fresh herbs (e.g., parsley or chervil)
approx 180 mg purine

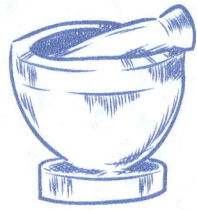

Instructions:

Cut the lemon in half after washing it in hot water. Half of the juice should be squeezed and rubbed onto the peel, and half of the remaining half should be cut into slices. Cut the chicken breast fillets in half horizontally after rinsing them under cold water and patting them dry. Turn in the flour and season with salt, pepper, and paprika powder. In a pan, heat 1 tbsp of olive oil. Cook the meat for 4–5 minutes on each side over medium heat. In the meantime, toss in the lemon wedges. Take the chicken and lemon out of the pan and set them aside.

Meanwhile, wash the asparagus, pat it dry, and trim the woody ends off. Cut the asparagus into 4–5 cm long sections. Garlic should be peeled and chopped finely.

In the same pan, heat the remaining oil and fry the garlic and asparagus bits.

Stir in the lemon juice, lemon zest, mustard, and stock, then bring to a boil for a few minutes. Reduce the heat to low and return the chicken breast fillet and lemon wedges to the pan to steep for a few minutes. Season with salt and pepper to taste.

Rinse the herbs, shake them off, and chop them coarsely. Sprinkle the lemon and asparagus chicken with a bit of salt and pepper.

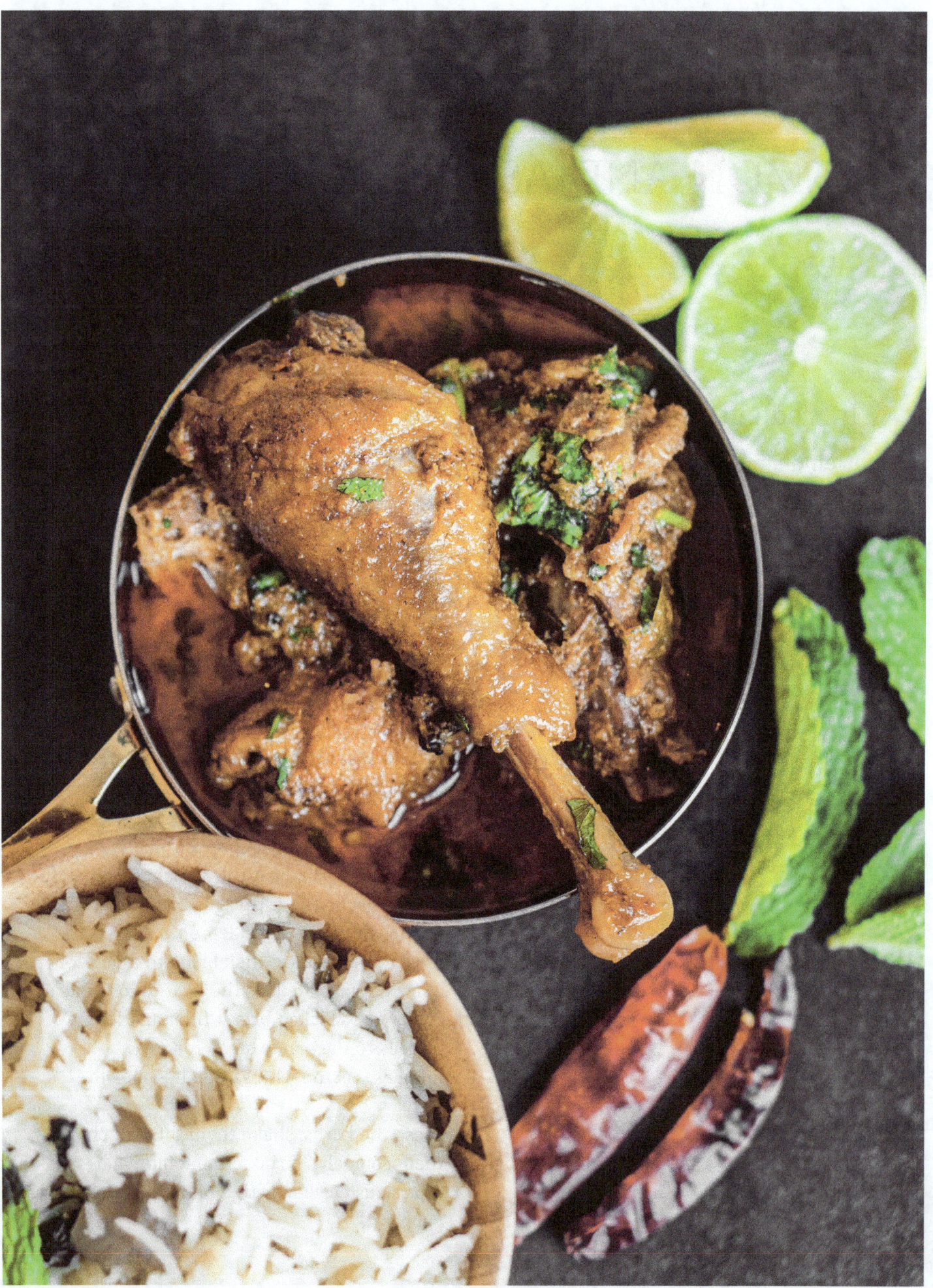

Servings: 4

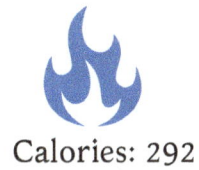
Calories: 292

Ready in 1 hour 45 min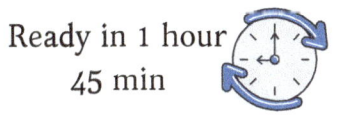

CHICKEN CASSEROLE

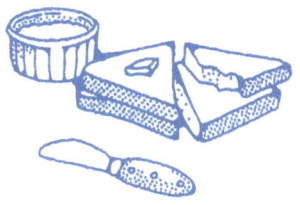

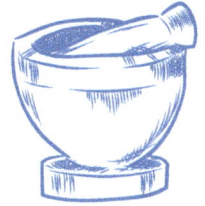

Ingredients:

6 fresh sage leaves
1 chicken (6 pounds)
3 tbsp olive oil (distributed)
1 ½ cup peeled and trimmed carrots,
1 cup peeled and cut turnips
2 cups peeled and halved fingerling potatoes
2 tbsp. fresh thyme, chopped
approx 175 mg purine

Instructions:

Preheat the oven to 190 C / 425 F. Under the skin of the chicken, put six lemon slices and sage leaves. Fill the cavity with the rest of the lemon. Tuck the wings under and tie the legs together with twine.

Coat the chicken with 1 tsp of oil. Place the chicken in a roasting pan and roast for 1 hour 15 minutes, or until an instant-read thermometer reads 165°F. Allow 15 minutes for the chicken to rest on a cutting board.

Meanwhile, make matchsticks out of root vegetables. Toss remaining oil and thyme with potatoes in a baking tray. Cook for 45 minutes, or until soft, stirring occasionally.

Take the chicken skin off. Take the lemons out of the cavity and throw them away. Serve with the vegetables.

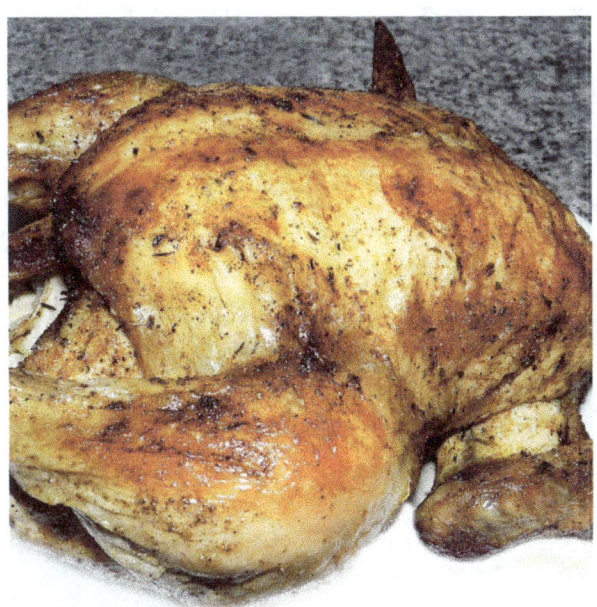

 Servings: 3

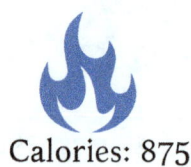 Calories: 875

 Ready in 1 hour 20 min

CHEESY CHICKEN BROCCOLI BAKE

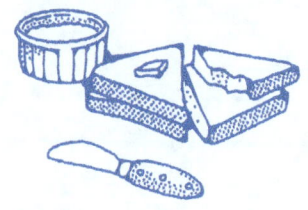

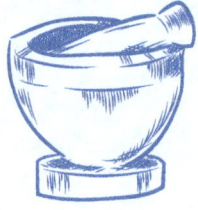

Ingredients:

1 big chicken breast
1 cup long-grain rice
¼ tsp black pepper
½ tsp onion powder
1 tbsp of cream
½ cup shredded cheddar cheese
2 cups broccoli, diced
1 ½ cups chicken broth
more cheddar cheese, for topping
approx 280 mg purine

Instructions:

Heat oven to 375°F (190°C).
In a casserole dish, combine rice, pepper, onion powder, cream, cheese, broccoli, and chicken broth. Mix until everything is combined.
Lay chicken on top of the rice mixture. Space evenly.
Cover with foil and bake for 50 minutes.
Take off the cover and top the chicken with more cheese. Bake uncovered for another 5 minutes or until the cheese is melted.

 Servings: 2

 Calories: 536

 Ready in 1 hour

ONE-PAN CHICKEN AND VEGGIES

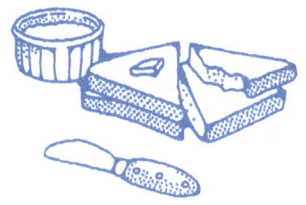

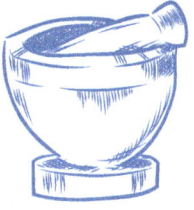

Ingredients:

2 boneless, skinless chicken breasts
1 large sweet potato, diced
1 head broccoli, or a large bag of broccoli florets
4 cloves garlic, minced
2 tbsp fresh rosemary
1 tbsp paprika
salt, pepper
2 tbsps olive oil
approx 240 mg purine

Instructions:

Line a baking sheet with aluminum foil. Layout the sweet potato, chicken breasts, and broccoli.

Evenly distribute the garlic, rosemary, paprika, salt, and pepper over the entire pan. Drizzle with olive oil.

Bake at 400°F (200°C) for 35-40 minutes (or until the internal temperature of the chicken reaches 165°F (75°C), and the juices run clear).

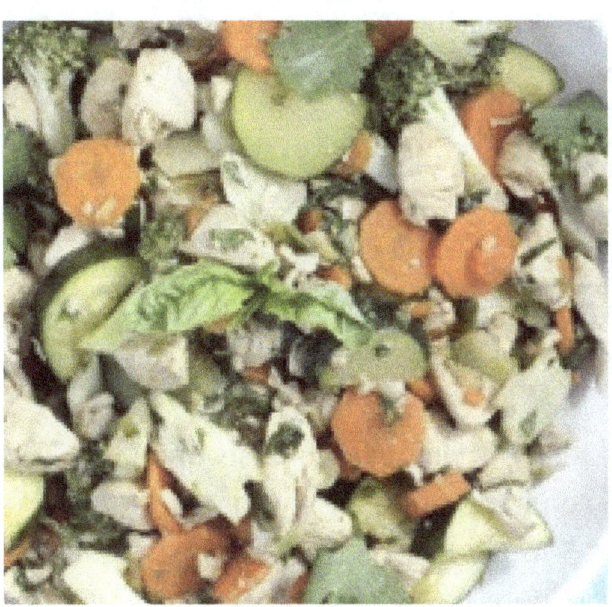

Servings: 2

Calories: 510

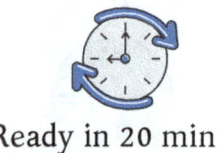
Ready in 20 min

CHICKEN WITH POTATOES

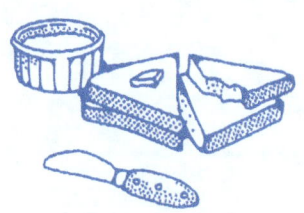

Ingredients:

1 ½ cup potatoes
1 cup tomatoes
1 bunch parsley
1 small onion
1 ½ cup breast fillet
cumin
4 tbsp of extra virgin olive oil
1 cup vegetable broth
approx 200 mg purine

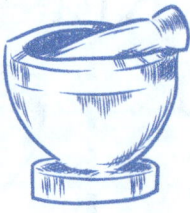

Instructions:

Boil the potatoes for 15-20 minutes, then drain. Meanwhile, wash the tomatoes, cut them in half, and strain out the seeds with your hands. Wash, dry, and chop the parsley. Onions should be peeled and chopped finely. Rinse the chicken breast fillet, pat dry, and slice thinly on an angle.

Place slices between two layers of cling film, flatten with a heavy pan or a meat tenderizer to form small schnitzels.

Heat a pan over high heat and fry the tomato halves without fat on the cut surface. Take tomatoes from the pan and put them aside. In the same pan, add 2 tbsps of oil, add the chicken and cook for 2-3 minutes on each side over medium. Remove chicken from the pan and keep them aside.

In the same pan, fry for 1-minute onion, then add tomatoes and chicken schnitzel.

Cook for another 2-3 minutes, then pour the broth over them. Season with salt, pepper, and parsley. Let boil on low heat for another 5 min.

Peel and dice the potatoes. In a second pan, heat the remaining oil and fry the potatoes for about 5 minutes on all sides over medium heat. Serve potatoes with chicken.

 Servings: 2

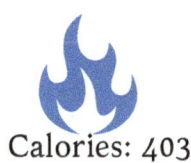 Calories: 403

 Ready in 1 hour

CHICKEN VEGETABLE SOUP

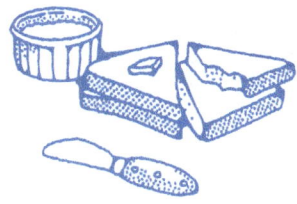

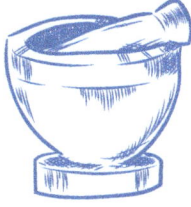

Ingredients:

2 chicken breasts
1 onion
1 soup vegetable bunch (plus other aromatic vegetables such as celery or onion)
2 lemons, tiny
1 tbsp olive oil
2 tsp. black pepper
1 leaf of bay
2 leaves of lime
2 garlic cloves
2 allspice berries
1 head of kohlrabi
3 waxy potatoes
½ cup peas
2 cups water
approx 225 mg purine

Instructions:

Clean the chicken breasts by rinsing them and patting them dry with paper towels.

Peel the carrots and parsley root from the soup vegetables. Trim the celery and leeks. One carrot, half a parsley root, half a celery stalk, and the leek greens, chopped. Pluck a few celery leaves, rinse them, and set them aside. Sear the onion halves in a pot coated with oil over high heat, then remove from the pan. Fry the chicken breasts in the same oil-coated pot over medium heat.

Combine the onion halves, chopped soup vegetables, and celery leaves in a large pot. Pour in about 2 cups of water and quickly bring to a boil. Add salt, peppercorns, bay leaf, lime leaves, cloves, allspice berries, and lemon slices. With the lid ajar, cook for about 20 minutes. Continue on the next page.

 Servings: 2   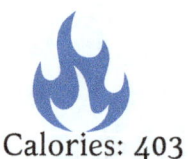 Calories: 403    Ready in 1 hour

CHICKEN VEGETABLE SOUP

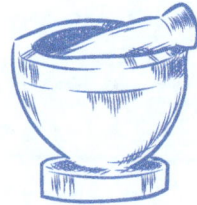

Instructions:

Continue from the previous page...

In the meantime, roughly chop the remaining soup vegetables. Potatoes and kohlrabi should be scrubbed and peeled before being cut into uniform sections.

Remove the chicken from the pot and place it on a plate.

Strain the cooking liquid into a separate pot using a fine sieve. To taste, season with salt and pepper.

Carry potatoes and remaining soup vegetables to a simmer over medium heat. The cooking time is about 15 minutes.

Cook for another 5 minutes after adding the peas and chicken.

Move the vegetables from the pot to plates with a slotted spoon. Pour a small amount of broth onto each plate. Place the chicken on top of the vegetable broth. Serve with the remaining chopped celery leaves.

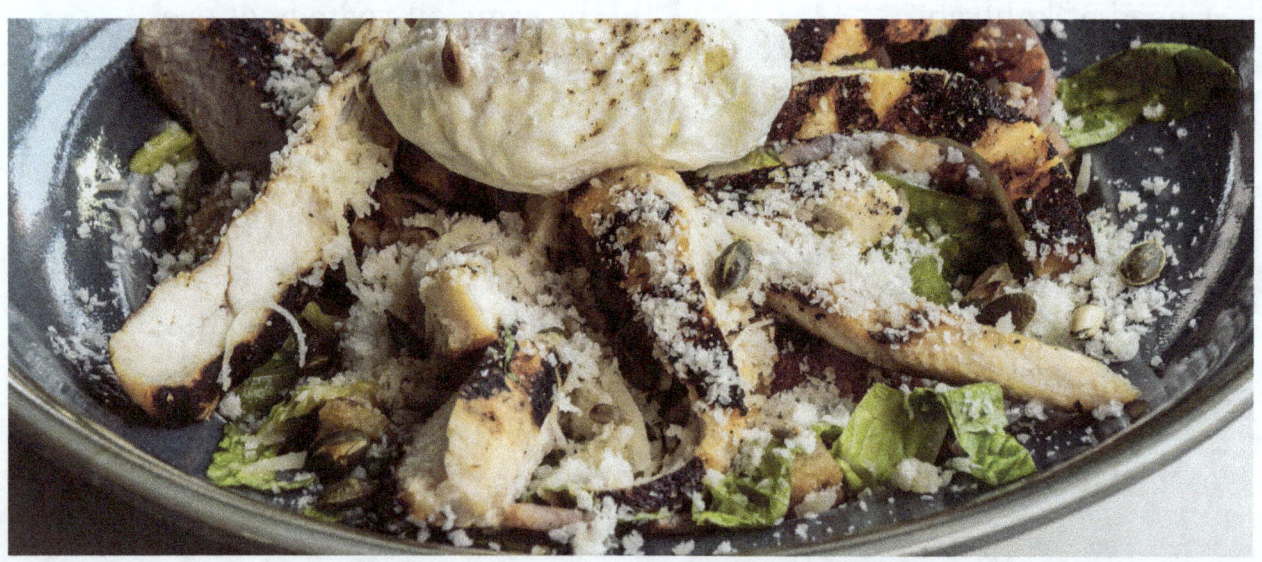

Servings: 2

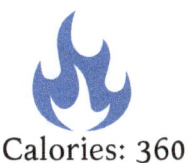
Calories: 360

Ready in 1 hour

CHICKEN AND LENTIL STEW

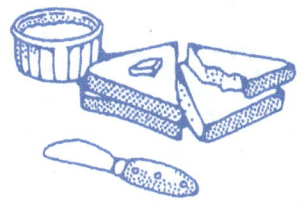

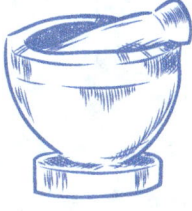

Ingredients:

1 cup dry lentils
2 cups chicken breast
1 tsp celery seed
1 tsp coriander
1 tbsp paprika
1 tbsp seasoning (Italian)
1 cup plain greek yogurt
(reserve a few tbsp to dollop on top at the end)
1/2 tiny orange, freshly squeezed
1 tbsp olive or coconut oil
1 chopped red onion
1/2 gallon coconut milk
1-quart chicken broth
a pinch of black pepper
garnish with parsley or cilantro
approx 350 mg purine

Instructions:

Boil 3 cups of water, add 1 cup dried green lentils and cook for 2 min. Turn heat off and let the lentils soak for 1 hour in the water. To make the chicken marinade, combine the chicken cubes with celery seed, 1/2 tsp coriander, paprika, and Italian seasoning in a mixing bowl add the greek yogurt, reserving a few tbsps to dollop on top at the end. Squeeze half an orange juice into the mixture and mix to incorporate both ingredients. Refrigerate for at least 10 minutes, up to 2 hours, with a lid or plastic wrap on top.

In the large cast iron dutch oven add 1 tbsp olive oil and marinated chicken and fry for 5 min, stirring occasionally. Toss in your chopped red onion, turn the chicken, and cook for another 5 minutes. Drain the lentils and add to the chicken, coconut milk, chicken broth, and salt/pepper. Stir to thoroughly mix, then cover and cook for 35 minutes, stirring occasionally.

Use a slotted spoon. Scoop the lentils and chicken into a bowl. Enjoy with a sprinkle of parsley and a dollop of plain Greek yogurt on top!

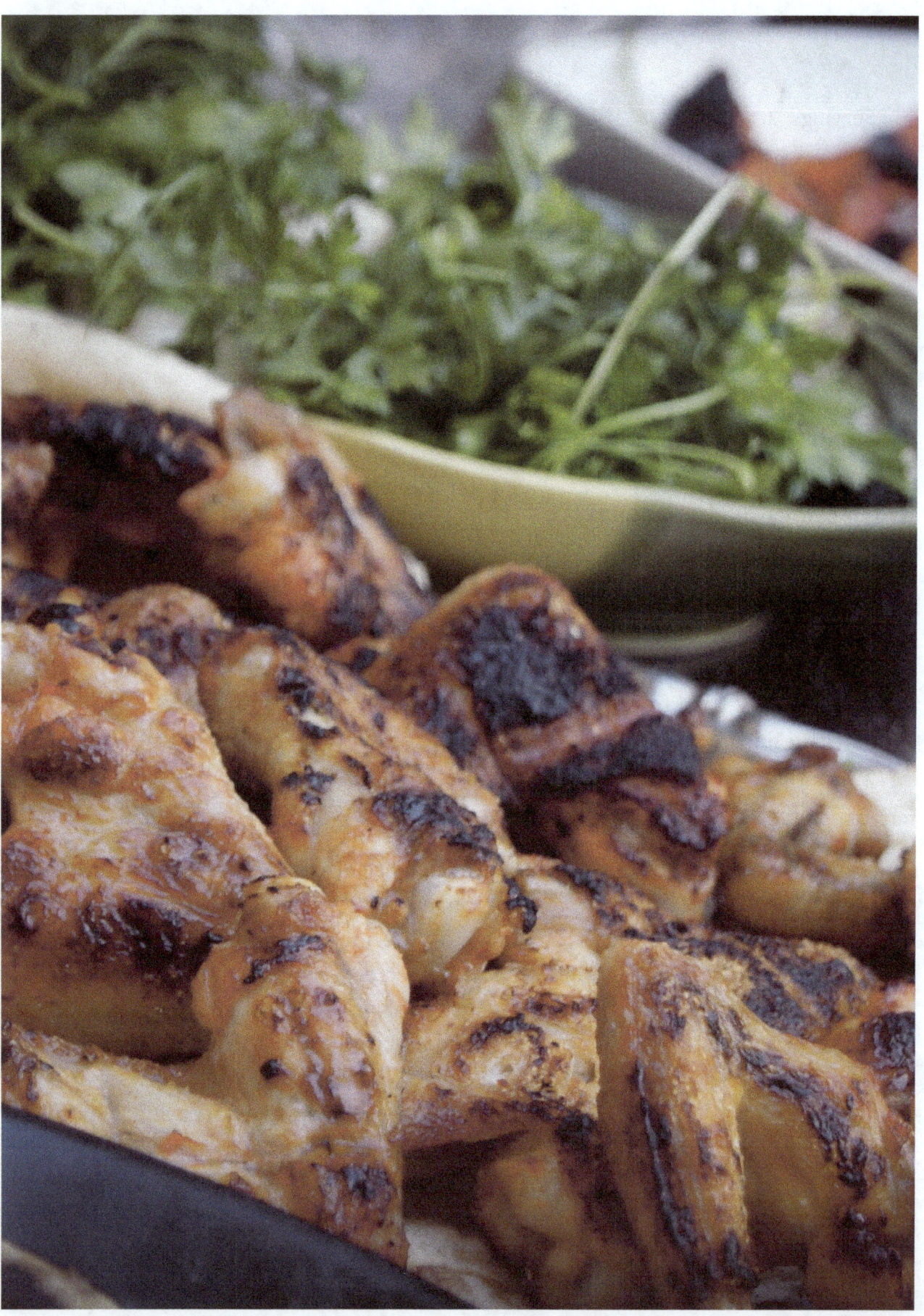

FISH

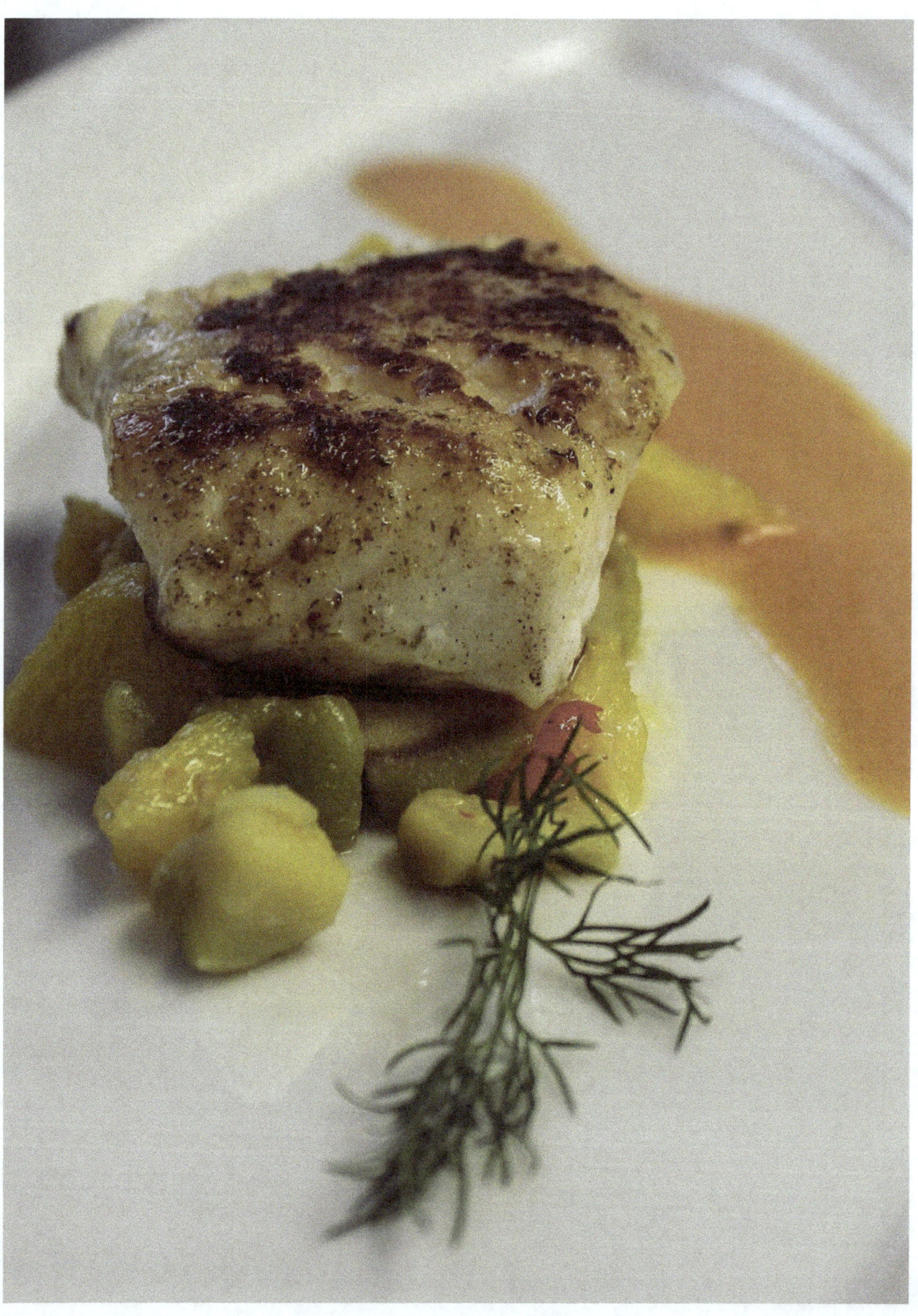

Servings: 2

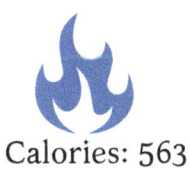
Calories: 563

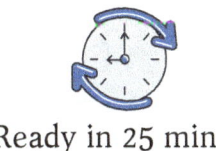
Ready in 25 min

SALMON ON FENNEL

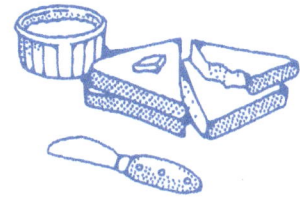

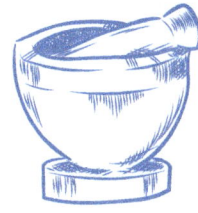

Ingredients:

1 red onion,
2 fennel tubers
2 or 3 tomatoes
2 thyme branches
2 tbsp walnut kernels
4 tbsp olive oil
salt
pepper cayenne
2 fillets of salmon
2 tsp provençal herbs
approx 180 mg purine

Instructions:

Peel the onion and cut it in half before slicing it into strips. Fennel should be cleaned and washed before removing the stalk, halving, and cutting into strips. Tomatoes should be cleaned, washed, and chopped. Pick the leaves off the thyme after it has been washed and dried. Chop the walnut kernels coarsely. Heat 2 tbsps of oil in a pan and cook the onion strips and fennel for 5 minutes over medium heat. Sauté for another 5 minutes with the nuts and tomatoes, add 2 tbsps of water and cook for another 5 minutes over low heat, sealed. Season with salt, pepper, thyme, and cayenne pepper to taste. Clean the salmon fillets by rinsing them, patting them dry, and seasoning them with salt. In a separate pan, heat the remaining oil and fry the salmon fillets for 3 minutes on both sides over medium heat, seasoning with herbs de Provence, salt, and pepper. On top of the vegetables, place the salmon fillet.

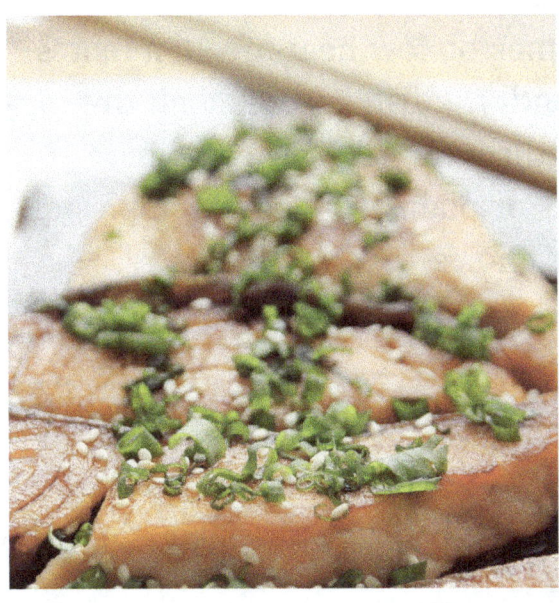

Servings: 4

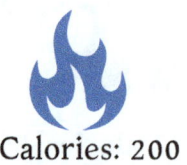
Calories: 200

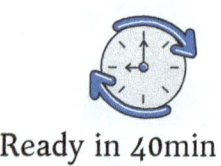
Ready in 40min

STEAMED SNAPPA

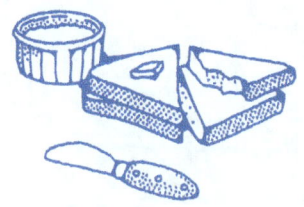

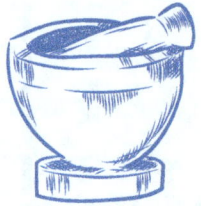

Ingredients:

½ cup of okra washed and trimmed
1 cup pumpkin peeled and cubed
4 medium snapper fish or another white fish on your choice
2 cloves of garlic crushed
1 onion thinly sliced
1 chopped tomato
½ tsp coarse black pepper
1 tsp ground coriander
1 bay leaf
2 whole pimentos
2 sprigs of thyme
scotch bonnet pepper
approx 170 mg purine

Instructions:

Season the fish with the scotch bonnet, garlic, black pepper, bay leaf, ground coriander, and thyme. This can be done in advance and left to marinate in the fridge overnight. Add the vegetables and a little water to a non-stick pan and heat gently for 5-7 minutes, then place the marinated fish on top of the vegetables and cover with a tight-fitting lid.

Simmer on low heat for 20 minutes or until the fish is cooked all the way through. Serve with boiled yams or plain rice and vegetables of your choice.

Servings 1

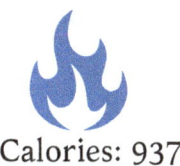
Calories: 937

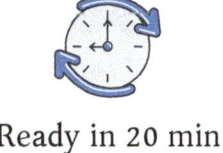
Ready in 20 min

AVOCADO LIME SALMON

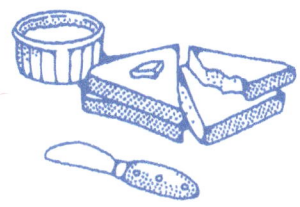

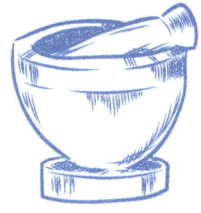

Ingredients:

6 oz skinless salmon(170 g)
1 clove garlic, minced
olive oil, to taste
salt, to taste
pepper, to taste
½ tsp paprika
for avocado topping:
1 avocado, chopped
¼ red onion, chopped
1 tbsp fresh cilantro, chopped
1 tbsp olive oil
salt, to taste, pepper, to taste
1 tbsp lime juice
approx 300 mg purine

Instructions:

Preheat the oven to 400°F (200°C). Line a baking sheet with parchment paper.
Rub the salmon with garlic, olive oil, salt, pepper, and paprika on the prepared baking sheet.
Bake for 10-12 minutes, until soft.
Make the avocado topping: In a small bowl, gently mix the avocado, red onion, cilantro, olive oil, salt, pepper, and lime juice. Don't overmix, or you'll break down the avocado.
Spoon the avocado topping over the salmon.

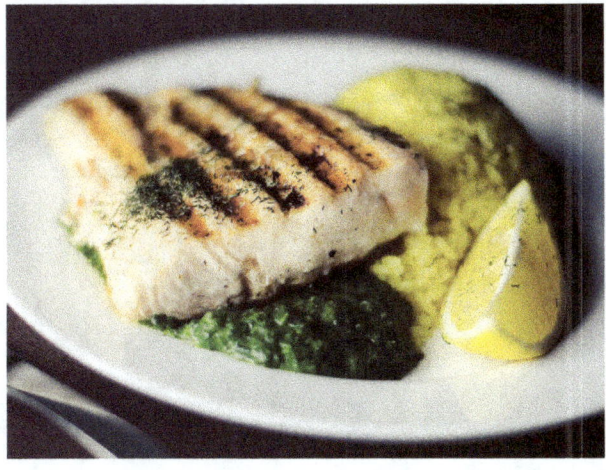

 Servings: 4

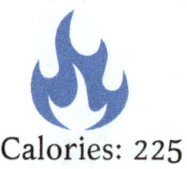 Calories: 225

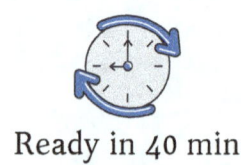 Ready in 40 min

SOLE IN OVEN

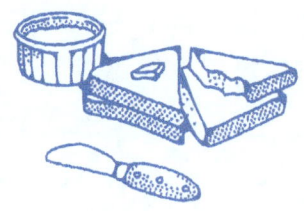

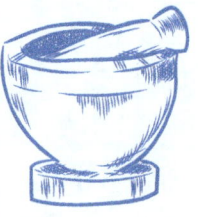

Ingredients:

4 fillets of sole fish
2 tbsp of olive oil
1 handful of parsley
1 tbsp of thyme,
1 sprig of rosemary
1 tbsp of marjoram
salt and pepper
2 cloves of garlic
juice of one lemon
1 lemon
approx 150 mg purine

Instructions:

Chop the garlic and parsley, add salt and pepper, marjoram, thyme. Put everything in a large dish with lemon juice and olive oil. Dip the fillets in the sauce on both sides and arrange them on a baking dish. Cut the lemon into wedges and dispose of them over the fillets. Add more parsley if you want. Bake in a preheated oven at 356F/180C for 20 minutes. Serve on a hot plate.

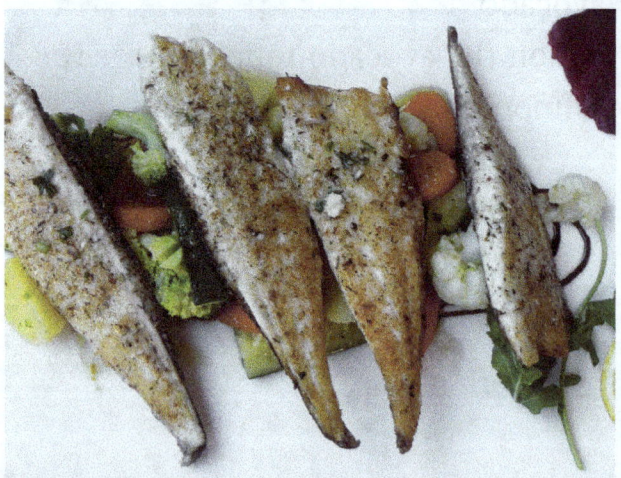

 Servings: 4

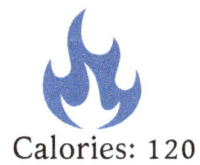 Calories: 120

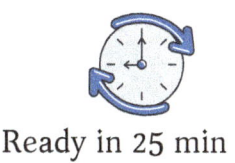 Ready in 25 min

BOILED SOLE

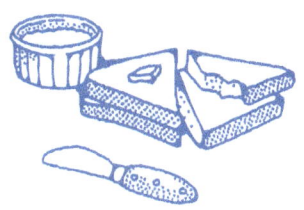

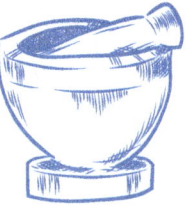

Ingredients:

4 fillets of sole
water
1 bunch parsley
1 bay leaf
1 tbsp of olive oil
coarse salt
lemon
approx 150 mg purine

Instructions:

Immerse the sole fillets in boiling water with parsley, bay leaf, extra virgin olive oil, and salt; then let it boil for about 15 minutes.
Drain them, put them on a plate, and season with oil, a little salt, and lemon.

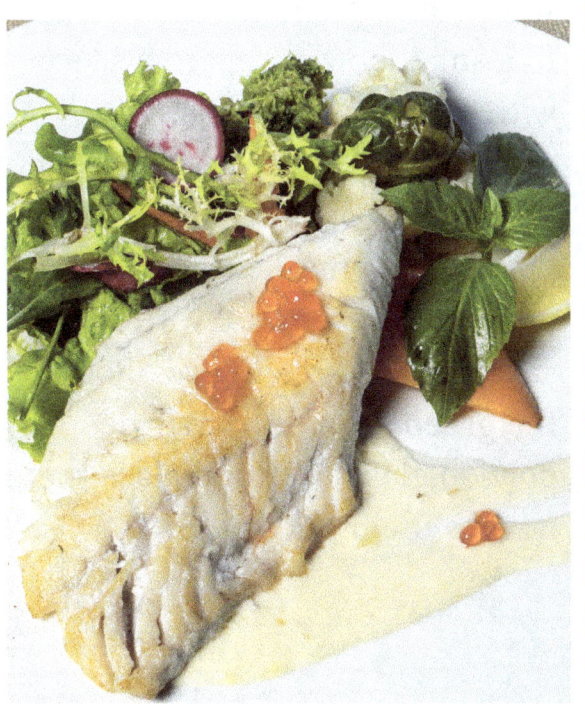

 Servings: 2

 Calories: 250

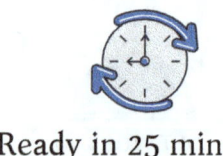 Ready in 25 min

MACKEREL WITH GREEN SAUCE

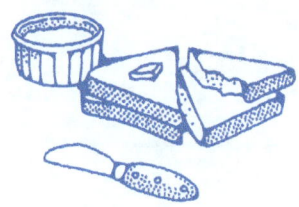

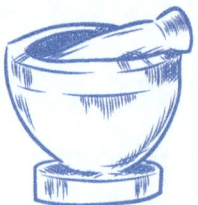

Ingredients:

1 medium-sized fresh mackerel
1 iceberg lettuce leaf
salt
black pepper
olive oil
1 clove garlic
1 handful of fresh parsley
lemon in juice
approx 160 mg purine

Instructions:

In a low and large pan, boil two fingers of water and add the whole mackerel, cover with the lid and let it cook 4/5 minutes. Turn off and let it cool.
For the green sauce: In a blender, mix the iceberg leaf, one tbsp water, and salt.
In a small bowl, prepare a sauce with oil, chopped parsley, quartered garlic, salt, black pepper, and a few drops of lemon. Arrange the mackerel steaks on a plate and season well with the sauce from a small bowl. Pour the green sauce into a single-portion glass bowl and place them next to the mackerel.

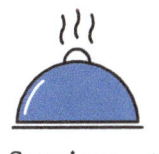
Servings: 4

Calories: 140

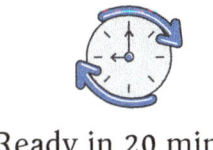
Ready in 20 min

COD IN WHITE SAUCE

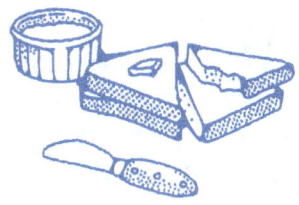

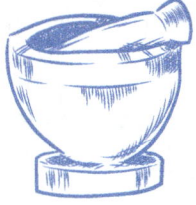

Ingredients:

4 cod fillets
5 tbsp of flour
olive oil
1 clove of garlic
1 lemon
2 tbsp of capers
10 olives
a handful of fresh parsley chopped
approx 130 mg purine

Instructions:

Flour the filets on both sides. Heat a little oil with a clove of garlic and brown it, careful not to burn the garlic.
Remove the garlic. Place the fish in the pan and fry them on both sides to take on a nice golden color.
Deglaze with the juice of a lemon, grate a little lemon peel, add capers and olives, and cook, taking care to keep the cod well moist and covered with the sauce.
Cover so that the sauce does not dry out too much, wait another minute or two and serve with fresh parsley.

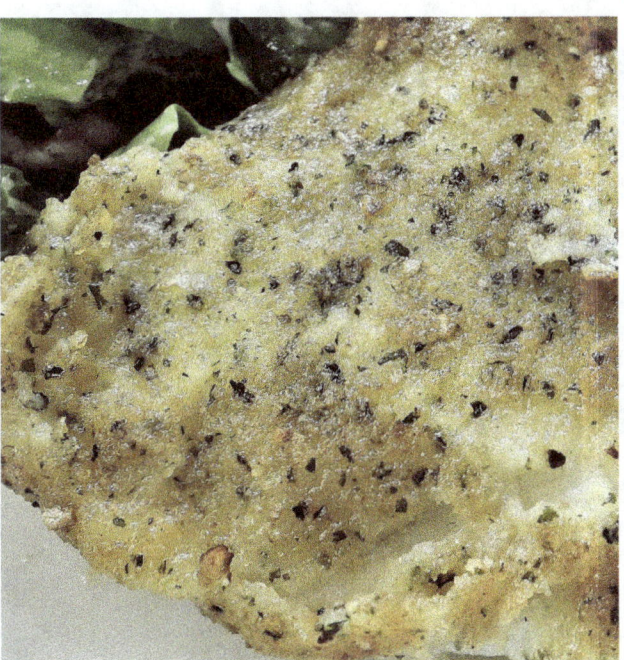

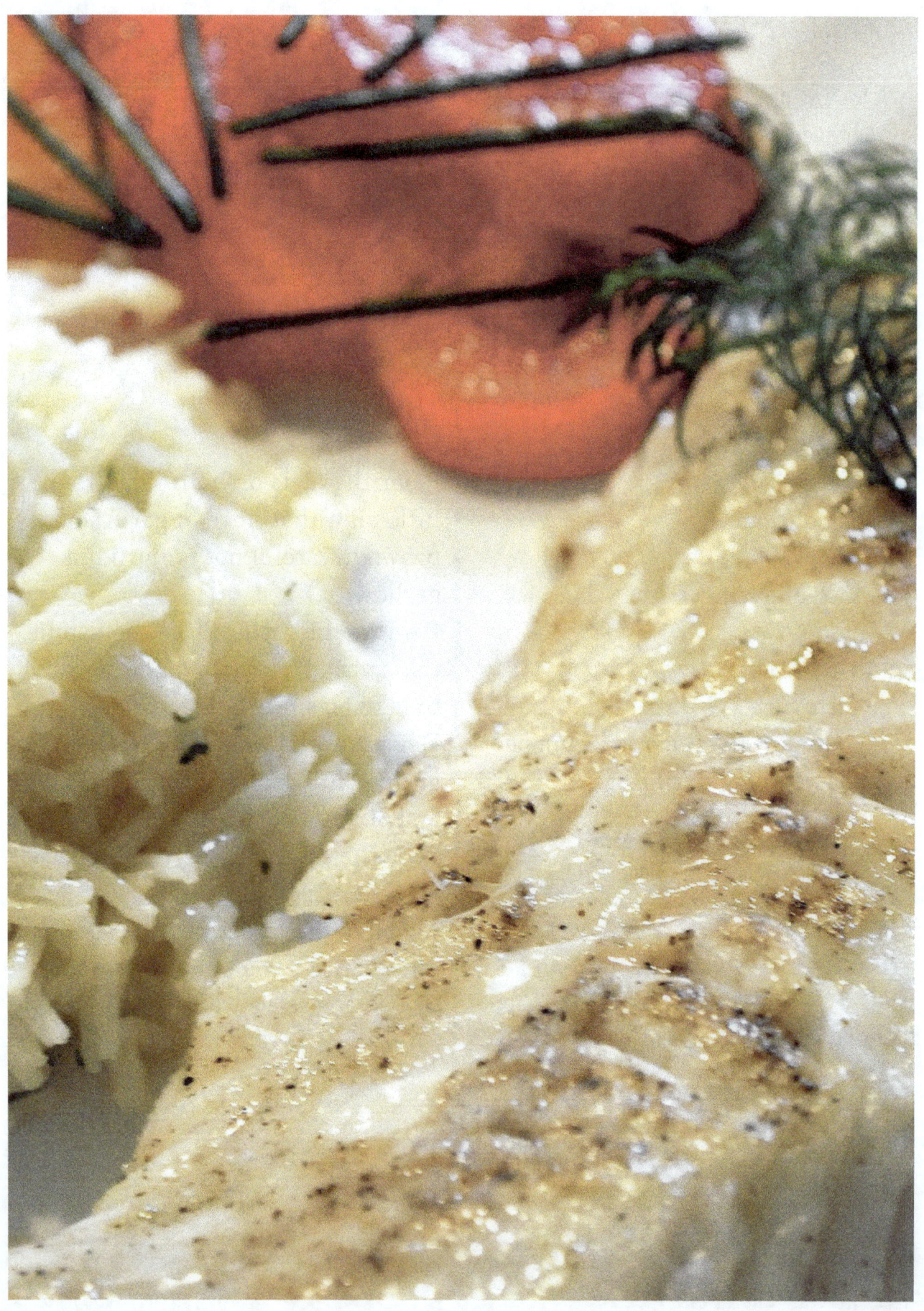

www.ingramcontent.com/pod-product-compliance
Lightning Source LLC
Chambersburg PA
CBHW081355080526
44588CB00016B/2505